Soap Making

A Complete Beginner's Guide to Natural Handmade

(Blend Natural and Organic Recipes, Master Cold, Hot, and Melt & Pour Methods)

Enrique Roderick

Published By **Tyson Maxwell**

Enrique Roderick

All Rights Reserved

Soap Making: A Complete Beginner's Guide to Natural Handmade (Blend Natural and Organic Recipes, Master Cold, Hot, and Melt & Pour Methods)

ISBN 978-1-7752619-8-8

No part of this guidebook shall be reproduced in any form without permission in writing from the publisher except in the case of brief quotations embodied in critical articles or reviews.

Legal & Disclaimer

The information contained in this book is not designed to replace or take the place of any form of medicine or professional medical advice. The information in this book has been provided for educational & entertainment purposes only.

The information contained in this book has been compiled from sources deemed reliable, and it is accurate to the best of the Author's knowledge; however, the Author cannot guarantee its accuracy and validity and cannot be held liable for any errors or omissions. Changes are periodically made to this book. You must consult your doctor or get professional medical advice before using any of the suggested remedies, techniques, or information in this book.

Upon using the information contained in this book, you agree to hold harmless the Author from and against any damages, costs, and expenses, including any legal fees potentially resulting from the application of any of the information provided by this guide. This disclaimer applies to any damages or injury caused by the use and application, whether directly or indirectly, of any advice or information presented, whether for breach of contract, tort, negligence, personal injury, criminal intent, or under any other cause of action.

You agree to accept all risks of using the information presented inside this book. You need to consult a professional medical practitioner in order to ensure you are both able and healthy enough to participate in this program.

Table Of Contents

Chapter 1: The Advantages Of Natural Soap Making 1

Chapter 2: Apricot Kernel Oil 22

Chapter 3: Activated Charcoal 41

Chapter 4: Cold Process Recipes 55

Chapter 5: Blue Lavender Soap 79

Chapter 6: Shea Butter Vanilla Coffee Soap 120

Chapter 7: Melt & Pour Recipes 137

Chapter 8: Lemon Pumice Soap 151

Chapter 9: The Essence Of Vegan Soap Crafting 156

Chapter 10: Vegan Soap Recipes 167

Chapter 11: Troubleshooting And Common Pitfalls 177

Chapter 1: The Advantages Of Natural Soap Making

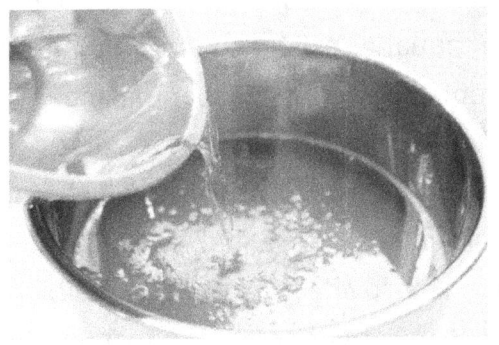

In an international more and more conscious of health, surroundings, and private nicely-being, the art work of natural soapmaking the usage of plant merchandise has emerged as a enjoyable and sustainable challenge for novices. Harnessing the advantages of vegan and herbal factors, this ancient craft offers numerous benefits that amplify beyond sincerely the introduction of excellent bars of cleaning soap. Let's delve into the ten compelling motives why embarking on a journey of herbal soapmaking may be every enriching and profitable for novices.

1. Environmentally Friendly: By retaining off artificial chemical materials that could harm aquatic existence and pollute water elements, herbal soapmaking places environmental friendliness first. Plant-primarily based substances which includes botanical oils, essential oils, and herbal colorants provide a greener possibility that reduces the environmental effect.

2. Gentle on Skin: Compared to the hard chemical substances determined in conventional soaps, vegan and plant-based totally components are generally kinder to the pores and skin. For beginners, crafting soaps with nourishing oils like coconut, olive, and shea butter guarantees a moisturizing and soothing enjoy for all pores and pores and skin sorts.

3. Customization and Creativity: Natural soapmaking offers a canvas for revolutionary expression. Beginners can check with diverse

scents, sun shades, and textures, infusing their soaps with a private contact. Ingredients like dried herbs, flower petals, and exfoliants permit for countless customization.

4. Aromatherapy Benefits: Utilizing crucial oils in natural soapmaking now not great offers quality fragrances however furthermore gives aromatherapy blessings. Beginners can discover one-of-a-type oils recounted for rest, rejuvenation, or stress consolation, enhancing the healing price in their creations.

five. Allergen Awareness: For people with sensitive skin or hypersensitive reactions, herbal soapmaking provides manage over substances, permitting novices to avoid commonplace allergens. This personalization guarantees that the cleaning soap fits person pores and pores and pores and skin desires with out triggering bad reactions.

6. Education on Ingredients: As novices dive into natural soapmaking, they grow to be greater knowledgeable approximately the

houses and advantages of various plant-based totally substances. With this elevated facts, they may be higher prepared to choose out greater realistic pores and pores and skin care regimens.

7. Minimalistic Approach: Natural soapmaking frequently promotes a far less tough way of life with the aid of encouraging the use of fewer substances, all of which serve specific functions. This minimalistic method resonates with novices searching for to declutter their exercises and embody aware consumption.

8. Sustainable Packaging: Beginners who need to incorporate sustainability might use inexperienced packaging materials that go along with the all-natural philosophy of their soaps. This holistic technique extends beyond soap introduction, contributing to a greener lifestyle.

nine. Connection to Nature: As novices interact with plant merchandise, they make bigger a deeper connection to the natural world. Harvesting herbs, infusing oils, and using earth-derived colorants instill a experience of awe and reverence for nature's splendor and assets.

10. Personal Fulfillment and Gifting: Crafting herbal soaps can be a supply of private accomplishment. The delight of creating a few factor tangible, coupled with the functionality to offer hand-crafted soaps to friends and circle of relatives, fosters a feel of satisfaction and strengthens interpersonal connections.

In surrender, the journey of herbal soapmaking the use of plant products offers a myriad of advantages that resonate deeply with beginners. From contributing to environmental properly-being and selling healthful pores and skin to fostering creativity and a connection to nature, this clever pursuit transcends the vicinity of crafting to embody holistic properly-being. As beginners embark on this enriching voyage, they not only create bars of cleaning soap however additionally include a aware and sustainable manner of life that echoes via each lather and fragrance.

List of Essential Ingredients

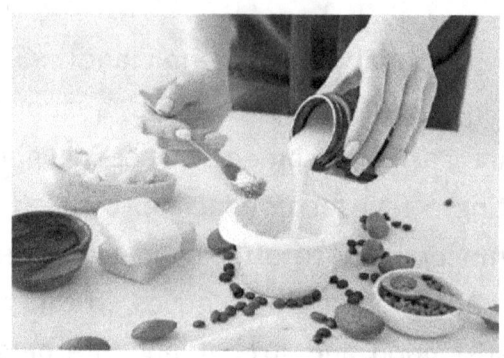

Necessary Equipment and Ingredients

SAFETY EQUIPMENT

Safety Goggles: It is important which you continually placed on a few form of protection gadget at the same time as coping with lye. To shield the eyes from splashes you want to location on safety goggles that cowl the eyes absolutely.

Safety Masks: Always wear a safety mask that is vapor proof in opposition to prevent breathing in risky lye fumes. It is suggested to shop for an industrial grade, heavy obligation masks that is rated N100 or P100 and for natural vapors in case you want to make essential cleaning cleaning soap over the long time.

Gloves: Your palms may be the closest to the lye as you parent, so you need to usually put on chemical resistant gloves, latex or nitrile gloves preferably. Preferably, use gloves with longer cuffs to ensure your wrists are protected well.

Appropriate Clothes and Shoes: To keep away from unintended splashes on the pores and pores and skin, continuously placed on lengthy-sleeved clothes and pants, preferably vintage clothes. Also wear closed-toe footwear to protect your toes.

OTHER EQUIPMENT

Digital Scale

The substances you may use in most soapmaking recipes are usually measured in metric weight (that is greater precise) in choice to volume. A scale can be gotten in maximum kitchen shops, you can get both a digital or guide scale, despite the fact that a digital scale is extra accurate. Get a scale which could measure as a minimum sixteen ounces., specially if you plan on making some of soap.

Stick Blender

Can also be called an immersion blender. When the oils are added to the lye answer, they need to be very well blended for emulsification to take location. A stick blender extensively reduces the amount of time the tracing way takes, from about 60 minutes to just a few mins. When out buying ensure you get one that has a stainless-steel shaft in choice to a plastic shaft.

Thermometer

The temperature of your elements desires to be monitored each earlier than and after mixing to make sure the method of saponification and emulsification is finished with none hitches. You can check the temperature the use of a tumbler candy thermometer or, higher but, a virtual thermometer.

Measuring Spoons and Cups

You can measure your elements, especially additives and colorants, using measuring spoons or cups. Make use of spoons and cups crafted from chemical and heat resistant fabric like chrome steel or plastic. However, note that plastic may be corroded by using the use of natural essential oils. Measuring cups also can be used for blending additives and colorants.

Heat Resistant Bowls

You want a large bowl or discipline for mixing the cleaning soap batter. They might be either glass, stainless-steel or plastic containers, simply make sure they may be chemical and warmth resistant. When blending lye water plastic or stainless-steel is most suitable as it cools faster than glass, and lye can etch glass boxes. Also, continuously use a bowl that is big than the quantity of cleaning soap batter you have got, with sufficient extra room left, to keep away from spills and other related injuries. Bowls and packing containers with handles and a pouring spout make it less complex to deal with and pour out from.

Small Glass Bowls/Cups

Essential oils without problems corrode plastic, so that they need to be treated, or maybe measured the usage of simplest glass cups or bowls. Shot glasses, canning jars and glass measuring cups additionally can be used to hold important oils.

Spoons, Spatulas and Whisks

A lengthy-dealt with chrome steel spoon may be used to stir and blend the batter, test for even as the batter consists of hint, and additionally can be used to create designs. Silicone or rubber spatulas are used to scrape out cleansing cleansing cleaning soap batter from the mixture discipline, and to create designs on the cleaning soap. Hand whisks or mixers are used for blending within the components and colorants. They aren't as powerful due to the fact the stick blender, so they may be used to gather and preserve the desired hint.

Cutter/Knife

Depending on the form of mold used, the cleansing soap also can moreover need to be reduce after unmolding. There are cleansing soap-cutters mainly designed for lowering cleaning cleaning soap, even a regular sharp knife that isn't always serrated will do the activity perfectly.

Slow Cooker

Additives like colorants and herbs are infused faster into the cleaning soap batter within the presence of heat. A gradual cooker allows to warm temperature the batter lightly as you introduce the components. You can also try this in a double boiler or a chrome steel saucepan over low warm temperature.

Coffee Grinder

(A mortar and pestle additionally may be used in location of this.) It may be used to pulverize herbs, colorants and different components, to lessen the chance of clumping and help mixture them resultseasily into the batter.

Molds

There are numerous styles of soap molds which can be to be had in lots of precise sizes, shapes and are fabricated from all types of cloth. So, one has a number of options to pick out from on the equal time as making cleansing cleaning soap, beginning from DIY cleaning cleaning soap molds, crafted from juice or milk or yogurt cardboard cartons, to extra favored molds made from plastic, wooden or silicone.

DIY Molds

There are masses of gadgets lying throughout the residence that you can use to make molds, items like waxed cardboard cartons that milk, yogurt or juice are generally presented in, plastic meals containers, and masses of others. They can all be used to make useful molds, but most times those substances can high-quality be used as speedy as because of the truth they get damaged via the oils in the cleansing soap batter, in particular cardboard made molds. When making DIY molds ensure that the soaps may be with out trouble removed from the mould, that is why glass and steel are not correct materials for making molds because of the truth the cleansing cleaning soap will maximum instances preserve on with it and be hard to do away with.

So, anything you pick out out to apply to make your mold, make sure that it has room for maneuverability to permit the cleaning soap to be eliminated. Cardboard made molds can be outcomes torn off to launch the cleansing soap, whilst molds made the usage of plastic substances can bend effortlessly to allow the cleaning cleaning soap to be removed. Importantly, while choosing what to use to make your mould use handiest what modified into used to maintain meals and unique constant materials. Also, make certain you operate heat water and cleaning soap to smooth them very well.

Loaf/Log Molds

They appear to be the most well-known shape of favored mildew sold. They is probably either silicone or wooden molds, and are available various sizes, however are in most instances square in form. Wooden molds appear stronger than silicone molds, but, at the same time as using wooden molds go for those mechanisms, like silicone inserts that could healthful into the mildew, or undersides that would slide out, or maybe elements that can be flipped open, which essentially assist to unmold soaps without troubles.

Silicone Molds

These have to now not be pressured with immoderate-density plastic molds, which can be more highly-priced and soap maintain on with plastic, making them more tough to put off from plastic molds. Silicone molds do not require any lining, are handy to art work with and make unmolding hundreds much much less complex even as in comparison to each wooden or plastic molds. However, the soaps want to be eliminated cautiously, the rims of silicone molds are softer and can with out problem dent the cleaning cleaning cleaning soap bar if not dealt with cautiously.

Using silicone molds calls for which you maintain temperatures low, due to the reality if the soap overheats the silicone fabric will go away scar marks at the cleansing soap. Although this does not affect how the final product feels or works.

LYE (THE MAIN INGREDIENT)

Lye is an essential element in cleansing cleaning cleaning soap making, if now not the maximum important. It is essential for the saponification approach to take location, in which it interacts with fats and oils to create cleansing soap, as emerge as previously referred to. Sodium hydroxide (NaOH) is normally known as lye, however, potassium hydroxide (KOH) is normally furthermore referred to as lye and is used to make liquid soaps and easy soaps.

Soaps are continuously made the use of lye in a few unspecified time in the destiny, so there may be no cleaning cleaning soap that can be termed lye unfastened. However, inside the soften and pour cleaning cleaning soap making approach the fat and oils are already saponified with lye to supply the soap base. So, the soften and pour method is recommended for parents which can be inquisitive about making home made soaps but are cautious about coping with lye.

During cleaning cleansing cleaning soap making, after all the components had been combined and poured right right into a mildew, the cleaning soap batter remains caustic due to the presence of lye. The harshness may be reduced after about 24 - 48 hours of saponification. However, the cleansing cleaning soap can burn the skin if used in advance than the saponification technique is complete, which typically takes approximately 4 - 6 weeks.

OTHER INGREDIENTS YOU NEED

BASE OILS

As has been said in advance, the shape of oil you operate in making your cleaning cleansing soap determines the form of cleaning cleaning soap you get, the way it feels, how hard or easy the cleaning cleansing soap can be, and different residences the cleaning soap has. This is because of the fact the fatty acid composition of the oil plays a top notch characteristic in the various tendencies which soaps own. It determines whether or not or now not your cleansing soap is conditioning and moisturizing the pores and pores and skin, whether or not or no longer or now not the cleaning cleansing soap produces huge bubbles and lathers properly, or how difficult and strong the cleansing cleansing soap is, or maybe influences the cleaning homes of soaps.

Most recipes generally combine at the least to three particular kinds of oils to provide the cleaning cleansing soap the popular nourishing and conditioning impact on the skin, mainly bathing soaps, facial soaps and luxury soaps. Laundry soaps as an opportunity do not require that lots idea, so most effective one or oils is normally sufficient to make a exquisite cleaning cleaning cleaning soap.

For example, soap made sincerely from coconut oil usually has awesome cleansing homes however can be pretty harsh on the pores and pores and skin, leaving it dry. The cleansing soap this is produced while first-rate olive oil is used, however, typically comes out to be very gentle because of the reality olive oil is well known for its emollient and conditioning houses. To seize up in this, a tougher oil needs to be mixed with olive oil, such that a cleaning cleaning soap that is nourishing and similarly tough and long-lasting can be made. This is why the traditional fats and oils typically utilized in cleansing cleaning soap making are olive oil.

Oils for Conditioning

Some of the oils that make contributions to the conditioning residences of soaps consist of castor oil, avocado oil, hemp seed oil, apricot kernel oil, cocoa butter, shea butter, olive oil, jojoba oil, sunflower oil, and cottonseed oil.

Among the oils used to create hydrating and nourishing soaps for the pores and pores and skin are cocoa butter, apricot kernel oil, argan oil, jojoba oil, castor oil, hazelnut oil, and neem oil.

Oils for Stable Lather

These oils, in conjunction with Jojoba oil, cocoa butter, shea butter, apricot kernel oil, argan oil, candy almond oil, and sunflower oil, are used to make soaps which have a strong lather and massive, lengthy-lasting bubbles.

Oils for Hard Soap

Any of the oils listed under can be added for your combination to reinforce your cleaning soap: Shea butter, cocoa butter, coconut oil, argan oil, palm kernel oil, and olive oil. Olive oil, which through itself produces easy cleaning soap, can solidify greater at the same time as coupled with different hardening oils.

Oils for Quicker Trace

To assist your cleaning soap batch obtain trace extra rapid, you may add cocoa butter, castor oil, shea butter, jojoba oil, palm kernel oil, or coconut oil.

Oils for Slower Trace

If you are producing a batch that requires sensitive and complex operations and you want the batch to hint slowly, you could use canola oil, hazelnut oil, sunflower oil, and soybean oil.

Butters

Typically, they provide soaps more frame and firmness, hydrating, conditioning, and increasing their shelf lives. They produce low-medium lather and characteristic low-medium cleaning abilties. Sal butter, mango butter, shea butter, kokum butter, and cocoa butter are some of them.

Chapter 2: Apricot Kernel Oil

It is a pores and pores and skin-satisfactory oil this is incredibly nourishing and hydrating. It smells nutty and is light in weight. Vitamins A, C, and E are sufficient, as well as linoleic and oleic acids. If applied in extra, it is able to make the cleaning soap easy and generates a ordinary, creamy lather with tiny bubbles. It is recommended to use an awful lot a whole lot much less apricot oil in your formulations ordinary—an awful lot much less than 10%—to boom the shelf existence of those soaps.

Substitutes: Hazelnut oil, Sweet Almond oil

Argan Oil

It originates from Morocco and is quite pricey. It feels silky and light-weight. It is moisturizing and has authentic conditioning capabilities. It is used to feature hardness to cleansing cleansing cleaning soap that comes out too easy, and it produces a robust rich lather. Argan oil is loaded with antioxidants and nutrients A and E. It have to make up to ten%

of the overall oils in recipes for cold manner cleaning soap.

Avocado Oil

It is a thick greenish oil complete of nutrients A, B, D and E and moreover palmitoleic and oleic acids. It has splendid conditioning homes and produces a medium creamy lather. Avocado oil has a bent to make soft soaps at the same time as used in greater, so it's far endorsed for use at 20% or lots much less of regular oils for your recipes. Its tendency to make gentle soaps makes it perfect for making conditioners, body butters, and lotions.

Substitutes: Sweet Almond oil, Chia Seed oil

Babassu Oil

Originates from Brazil and is taken into consideration an tremendous alternative for coconut and palm kernel oils, because of its similarity to the ones oils. It has comparable cleaning houses and adds hardness to bloodless method cleaning cleaning soap recipes. However, it's miles extra fast absorbed into the pores and pores and skin than coconut oil and is lighter and kinder to the pores and pores and skin. It is immoderate in food plan E, phytophenols, and numerous precise antioxidants, and additionally lauric and myristic acid which is answerable for producing immoderate lather and bubbles.

Substitutes: Coconut oil and palm kernel oil

Beeswax

In order to increase the hardness of cleaning soap recipes that have a propensity to reveal out gentle, it is added in cold technique soap recipes, up to eight% of fashionable oils. It hurries up trace and stays completely melted at temperatures above a hundred and fifty°F, as such you may want to art work rapid at such excessive temperatures while the use of beeswax in your recipe. Beeswax does not go through saponification absolutely and so gives the cleaning soap a herbal moisturizing functionality.

Substitutes: Cocoa butter

Canola Oil

It is cheap and can be used as an much less costly alternative to natural olive oil. It is moisturizing and produces a low and creamy lather. Canola oil takes longer to trace and can be used to slow down the price of saponification in cleansing soap recipes that consist of sensitive and complex strategies like swirls that take a longer time to complete.

Substitutes: Olive oil, Rice Bran oil

Castor Oil

It is a golden-yellow liquid, very immoderate in ricinoleic acid, a fatty acid with robust recovery houses. Rashes and severa different pores and skin illnesses are generally handled with it. It is moisturizing with appropriate skin conditioning houses. You can burn up to five% on your cleansing soap recipes, but not more than 10%, above which may also moreover bring about a completely tender and sticky cleansing cleaning soap bar. Castor oil is thought for rushing up hint in cleaning soap recipes. It offers a wealthy creamy lather with immoderate robust bubbles.

Substitutes: None

Cocoa Butter

It can be very moisturizing and has correct conditioning homes. It does now not saponify completely and so transmits its herbal moisturizing homes to the cleansing soap. Cocoa butter is difficult at room temperature; as a result, it enables to add hardness to cleaning cleaning soap. It creates a thick, regular lather and gives cleansing cleansing soap a expensive experience. Vitamin E and antioxidants are sufficient. Cocoa butter need for use at 15% or lots less in bloodless technique recipes, using an excessive amount of will supply a cleaning cleaning soap that is cracked, crumbly and hard, that produces low lather.

Substitutes: Shea butter, Mango butter, Beeswax

Coconut Oil

The maximum common coconut oil sold in stores is the handiest that melts at seventy six°F, there can be a second version that melts at ninety two°F. They each have the same SAP fee and bring the identical form of soap. In this ebook all recipes that embody coconut oil makes use of the 76-degree coconut oil. Due to its wonderful cleaning capabilities, coconut oil has the capability to burn up the pores and pores and skin of its herbal oils, leaving it dry. It gives a tough cleaning soap that produces excessive lather with masses of bubbles. It may be used as a whole lot as 30% in cleaning soap recipes, despite the fact that it's also endorsed to apply an awful lot much less than 20% if you have touchy skin. Coconut oil can really be used as much as forty% in a cleansing cleansing cleaning soap recipe, however you have to compensate through growing the superfat content cloth of the recipe.

Substitutes: Babassu oil, Palm Kernel oil

Grapeseed Oil

It is a light-weight oil that feels silky to touch and does now not leave a greasy after feeling at the same time as done to the skin. Linoleic acid, omega-6 fatty acids, and antioxidants are enough in it. It is moisturizing with incredible conditioning homes and offers soaps that produce creamy robust lather. It is right for pimples because of its astringent assets. It may be used up to ten% in bloodless tool soap recipes.

Substitutes: Hazelnut oil, Olive oil

Hazelnut Oil

It is an amber colored, mild-weight oil that is outcomes absorbed into the pores and pores and skin. It has remarkable moisturizing and cleaning functions and yields a cleansing soap that offers a stable bubbly lather. It is immoderate in oleic acid and slows down the charge at which a cleaning soap reaches trace. This makes it an first-rate oil for soaps that contain complex techniques that take time. It can be used up to 15% in cleansing cleaning soap recipes.

Substitutes: Grapeseed oil, Hemp Seed oil, and Apricot Kernel oil

Hemp Seed Oil

It produces cleaning soap that is exceedingly hydrating with a skinny, creamy lather and is a greenish-slight oil this is excessive in vitamins A and E. Due to its low shelf existence, soaps made with it need to use up in advance than six months. You can expend to 10% in bloodless manner recipes, despite the fact that during case you need to make a cleaning soap bar that lasts longer than six months you then clearly want to use an lousy lot an awful lot less than 5% of popular oils.

Substitutes: Avocado oil, Hazelnut oil

Jojoba Oil

It is a liquid wax with similar chemical composition to the pores and skin natural oil - sebum. It is proper for prolonged-lasting soaps because of the fact it is noticeably solid and has a extended shelf lifestyles. Jojoba oil is without difficulty absorbed into the pores and skin, it does now not saponify absolutely, and yields soaps which might be moisturizing and conditioning, with rich sturdy lather. It may be used up to 10% in your recipes. Too an lousy lot Jojoba oil in a cleaning soap batch can bring about low lather.

Macadamia Nut Oil

This skinny oil is rich in oleic acid, omega-6 and omega-3 fatty acids, and antioxidants. It has a slight nutty perfume and is with out trouble absorbed thru the pores and skin. It gives soaps more firmness and produces a nutritious, conditioning cleaning cleansing cleaning soap with a creamy lather. It should make up to 15% to twenty% of the entire oils to your batch of cleaning soap.

Mango Butter

At room temperature it's far a soft butter which melts while it encounters the pores and skin. It is fairly moisturizing and yields a difficult bar this is conditioning and nourishing to the pores and pores and skin, with wealthy creamy lather. This makes it useful for making facial soaps, and for dry pores and pores and skin. It is excessive in antioxidants and nutrients A and C. You can use mango butter up to twenty% of stylish oils in cold approach recipes.

Substitutes: Cocoa butter, Shea butter

Neem Oil

It has a exceptional earthy, musky fragrance to it; however, it's miles widely known for having anti-bacterial, anti-inflammatory, and antifungal results. It has long been used as an insect repellent, skin calming, and a remedy for some pores and skin issues like athlete's foot. It yields a hard lengthy-lasting cleaning soap bar that is very conditioning and moisturizing, giving a creamy stable lather. Neem oil is proper for touchy pores and skin and for pimples. It may be used as much as five% in cleansing cleaning soap recipes. If delivered in more, the consequent cleaning cleansing soap bar may additionally have a mild odor.

Olive Oil

The oldest and most used base oil for producing cleansing soap is that this one. Pure or virgin olive oil may be very conditioning and moisturizing. However, it gives a smooth cleaning soap with low cleansing capability and low lather, that takes an prolonged time to trace. These soaps are mild and slight, perfect for sensitive pores and pores and skin, infants and those with positive pores and skin conditions. It can be used as masses as one hundred% in cleaning cleaning cleaning soap recipes (Castile cleaning soap). Pure/virgin olive oil became utilized in all recipes that encompass olive oil in this e-book.

Pomace olive oil is a thick, greenish grade of olive oil that offers a harder but similar cleaning cleansing soap bar this is slight and moisturizing. It does no longer saponify absolutely and takes a miles shorter time to hint than herbal olive oil. Olive oil in big is complete of antioxidants like polyphenols and nutrients E.

Substitutes: Grapeseed oil, Canola oil, and Rice Bran oil

Shea Butter

It imparts a creamy, opulent enjoy to cleaning cleaning soap, is with out issues absorbed with the aid of the usage of manner of the pores and pores and skin, and aids in hardening a batch of smooth cleaning soap. It produces a moisturizing and conditioning cleansing soap that has a stable lather, is long-lasting, and is ok in fatty acids, nutrients A, and E. Shea butter could make cleansing cleaning cleaning soap hint extra fast and make up to fifteen% of the overall oil content material cloth for your cleansing cleaning soap formulations.

Substitutes: Cocoa butter, Mango butter

Sunflower Oil

It is a light-weight reasonably-priced oil, full of essential fatty acids and nutrients E. It gives a moisturizing and conditioning soap, with stable lather, pleasant for dry skin. It slows down how quick a batch of cleansing cleaning soap lines. Sunflower oil may be used up to 20% of popular oils on your recipe, which includes more will yield a mild cleaning cleansing soap bar.

There are kinds of sunflower oil which can be provided in stores, sunflower oil this is high in oleic acid and sunflower oil this is excessive in linoleic and linolenic acids. It is normally encouraged that you use the excessive oleic sunflower oil in cleansing cleaning soap making, that is because of the truth they've got an extended shelf existence than one-of-a-type sunflower oils immoderate in linoleic and linolenic acids.

Generally, oils with immoderate linoleic and linolenic content material generally tend to transport rancid more speedy, so soaps made the use of them should have a shorter shelf lifestyles as compared to soaps made the usage of oils immoderate in oleic acid.

Substitutes: Safflower oil, Olive oil

Sweet Almond Oil

Almond Oil Sweet Lightweight sweet almond oil has brilliant moisturising abilties. It is a amazing supply of fatty acids and nutrients A, D, and E, has a golden-yellow tint, and is quickly absorbed through the pores and pores and pores and skin. It is right for skin sorts which may be touchy, dry, inflamed, or flaky. A moderate cleansing cleaning soap made with candy almond oil has suitable moisturizing and conditioning traits that create an extended lasting lather. It is effects saponified and can be implemented up to 20% in bloodless way recipes.

Substitutes: Avocado oil, Apricot Kernel oil, Chia Seed oil

1. NATURAL ADDITIVES & COLORANTS

Natural soaps genuinely require simply the three number one additives, fat and oils, lye and water. Any specific detail apart from those three are not in fact critical to make a cleansing cleaning soap, within the genuine experience of the word. Natural additives are delivered to cleaning soap to provide it person, a completely specific revel in, colour, layout or perfume.

Natural components can be used to make the cleaning soap extra appealing, and upload extraordinary excellent trends like moisturizing, conditioning, exfoliating or nourishing homes on your cleansing cleaning cleaning soap batch. For example, a cleaning soap bar can be made more bubbly by using including honey to it. Other components like aloe, coconut milk, avocado, clay and goat milk, which might be naturally rich in vitamins, antioxidants and distinct minerals add moisturizing and nourishing homes to cleaning soap.

Coffee ground and oats can be used to make exfoliating soaps, while plant life of plants like calendula, lavender and rose can be used as ornament on cleansing cleaning soap bars. Herbs like chamomile, peppermint, green tea, and comfrey additionally add exfoliation homes to soaps. These herbs, being wealthy in vital minerals and nutrients, additionally upload nourishment, and are conditioning to the pores and skin.

Just as precise additives upload particular homes whilst brought to cleansing soap, so additionally, they behave in every other manner. Some components have a tendency to make cleaning cleansing cleaning soap come to hint faster, at the equal time as others gradual down the machine of hint. Some will change coloration while the soap is completely saponified, while a few will significantly growth the temperature of the combination at the same time as brought. So, you need to be privy to which additive you're along with, and the way you control the mixture afterwards.

Honey

It is a humectant, and an effective antimicrobial agent. Honey consists of natural sugars and antioxidants, which makes it better than regular sugar. Sugar in cleaning cleaning soap will increase lather production and makes the cleaning soap bubblier. Ideally, you upload 1 tablespoon of honey in keeping with pound of cleaning cleaning soap.

Dried Herbs/Flowers

Herbs together with lemongrass, peppermint, lavender, spearmint, calendula, basil, chamomile, and rosemary can be added to cleaning cleansing soap for exfoliation. It is major to apply dried and crushed herbs, approximately 1 teaspoon regular with 450g of your preferred base oils earlier than mixing with the lye answer.

Most vegetation and herbs, except calendula, will flip brown, or maybe black whilst introduced to cleansing cleaning soap at hint. Add the dried plants, for decoration, to the top of the cleaning cleansing cleaning soap before it devices to keep away from this.

Seeds

Seeds like chia seeds, cumin, strawberry, cranberry, blueberry, cardamom, or raspberry seeds may be brought to cleansing cleaning soap for exfoliation. Before blending the bottom oils with the lye solution, you can upload your preference seeds to the bottom oil, up to at least one teaspoon in line with 900g of base oil.

Clays

Clays like kaolin, zeolite, bentonite or pink clay have suitable cleaning houses, and are moderate exfoliants. They upload colour to cleaning cleansing soap and are true detoxifiers. The form of clay you upload will rely on what you need in your cleaning soap.

You can add up to 1 teaspoon consistent with 450g of base oils, including greater can supply a darker color, on the equal time as including tons less a lighter colour. Clay also may be introduced without delay to lye water to attract out the colour from the clay.

Chapter 3: Activated Charcoal

Activated charcoal has extremely good cleaning powers and is a extraordinary detoxifier. Though they make black or gray soaps, they do no longer stain and in fact supply white lather. Such soaps are tremendous for psoriasis, zits, and eczema. It can be used up to at least one teaspoon normal with 450g of base oils.

Coffee Ground

Adding floor espresso to cleansing cleaning soap yields a calming and exfoliating cleansing cleaning soap with a darkish brown shade. Coffee ground can be delivered up to one tablespoon consistent with pound (450g) of base oils. You may additionally want to every add it to base oils earlier than blending with lye solution or upload it right now to the lye solution.

Oatmeal

Oatmeal may be delivered entire or floor to cleansing cleaning soap to provide it moisturizing and exfoliating homes. Oatmeal is definitely calming, soothing, and nourishing to the pores and skin. Oatmeal cleaning cleansing soap can be used to address acne, darkish circles and wrinkles. You can expend to at the least one tablespoon of oatmeal steady with 450g of base oils, earlier than blending with the lye solution.

COLORANTS

In addition to in conjunction with nutritive and exfoliation homes to cleansing cleaning soap, additives are also used to characteristic color and different ornamental elements to cleansing cleansing soap. Such components are referred to as colorants.

Coffee brew, floor cloves, floor cinnamon and cocoa powder can be used to feature brown coloration to soap. Black or grey is gotten from activated charcoal, blue from indigo root or woad powder. You should make yellow colored cleansing soap the usage of floor turmeric, ground ginger, floor calendula plant life and saffron. Orange from Moroccan clay, pumpkin puree, tomato puree, carrot juice, paprika, and annatto seeds. Green from parsley leaf, spirulina powder, comfrey leaves, nettle leaf, liquid chlorophyll, dandelion leaf, and burdock leaf. Red from madder root, pink from rose clay, and purple from alkanet root powder.

Colorants may be brought to cleaning soap thru three important strategies. You can add them right away into the lye water and stir; you may moreover add the colorant at trace; or by way of way of way of first developing an oil infusion the usage of the colorant, then upload the oil infusion into the cleansing cleaning soap. The oil infusion method is commonly accomplished to avoid speckles within the cleaning soap.

When including colorants at hint, allow the cleaning soap to reap a light trace then scoop out a touch proper right into a discipline or measuring cup. Ensure there are not any lumps thru whisking inside the colourant earlier than which encompass it to the quantity that modified into scooped out. After whisking, upload the element decrease returned into the cleansing soap batch and blend very well to aggregate the coloration completely into the batch.

An oil infusion can be created via first together with about 2 ounces of colorant right into a dry, easy canning jar. Eight oz.. Of olive oil must be delivered to the jar, then it must be carefully closed. In a cool and dry cabinet, allow to infuse into oil for about five weeks, on the same time as from time to time shaking the jar to combine oil and colorant. This is called cold infusion.

In warm infusion, the coloration is drawn out a bargain quicker, normally taking much less than half-hour. To make a warmness infusion, set a slow cooker or pot full of water on a choice, turn the warmth to medium if using a gradual cooker, and coffee if the use of a pot. Put the jar inside the water and warmth for about 20 mins, once in a while shaking the jar.

Strain the infusion at the same time as it is ready.

When including an infusion, the quantity of olive oil on your recipe may be reduced with the resource of way of the quantity of oil infusion brought. So, if 10 oz.Of olive oil modified into earlier than the whole lot used within the recipe, and a couple of oz.. Of the infusion become used, then the olive oil must be reduced to eight oz..

Various colorants can be brought in more than one way into the cleansing soap; but, high-quality colorants may also require a specific addition approach to get the pleasant and simplest shade from them.

Added to Lye Water

Brewed espresso (2 teaspoons in keeping with 450g of cleansing soap)

Spirulina powder (½ teaspoon in step with 450g of cleaning cleansing cleaning soap)

Paprika (1 teaspoon consistent with 450g of cleaning cleaning soap)

Ground Calendula vegetation (¼ cup constant with 450g of cleansing cleaning cleaning soap)

Madder root powder (2 teaspoons in line with 450g of cleansing soap)

Indigo powder (1 teaspoon in line with 450g of cleansing cleaning soap)

Rose clay (2 teaspoons in step with 450g of cleaning soap)

Added at Trace

Activated charcoal (1 teaspoon according to 450g of soap)

Cocoa powder (1 tablespoon in keeping with 450g of soap)

Paprika (1 teaspoon consistent with 450g of cleaning cleansing soap)

Ground cinnamon (2 teaspoons steady with 450g of cleaning cleaning cleaning soap)

Spirulina powder (½ teaspoon in step with 450g of cleaning soap)

Madder root powder (2 teaspoons in keeping with 450g of soap)

Rose clay (2 teaspoons consistent with 450g of soap)

Liquid chlorophyll (1 teaspoon normal with 450g of cleaning cleaning soap)

Moroccan clay (1 teaspoon in line with 450g of cleansing cleaning soap)

Alkanet root powder (½ teaspoon consistent with 450g of cleaning soap)

Added by using the usage of Oil Infusion

Alkanet root powder (zero.Five ouncesof oil infusion In line with 450g of cleansing cleansing soap, in location of ollve oil in recipe)

Wood powder (0.Five ouncesof oil infusion in step with 450g of cleaning soap, in place of olive oil in recipe)

Parsley leaf (zero.Five ounces. Of oil infusion consistent with 450g of cleansing soap, in location of olive oil in recipe)

Saffron (0.Five ozof oil infusion in step with 450g of cleansing cleaning soap, in location of olive oil in recipe)

Ground turmeric (0.Five oz.. Of oil infusion in step with 450g of cleansing soap, in area of olive oil in recipe)

Ground ginger (1 ounce of oil infusion constant with 450g of cleansing cleansing soap, in place of olive oil in recipe)

Alfalfa (zero.Five ouncesof oil infusion in step with 450g of cleaning cleaning soap, in place of olive oil in recipe)

Dandelion leaf (zero.Five ounces. Of oil infusion regular with 450g of cleaning cleaning cleaning soap, in location of olive oil in recipe)

Burdock leaf (zero.Five ounces.. Of oil infusion consistent with 450g of soap, in vicinity of olive oil in recipe)

Annatto seeds (1.Five oz. Of oil infusion consistent with 450g of cleaning soap, in place of olive oil in recipe)

2. ESSENTIAL OILS

Anyone who alternatives up a brand new cleansing cleaning soap bar almost typically right away brings it as an lousy lot as their nostril to heady scent it, and maximum instances they try this without questioning that it can be defined as a reflex movement. So, no question the perfume of a cleaning cleaning soap bar, in addition to unique satisfactory trends, makes it more appealing to whoever wants to use it.

In cleansing soap making, crucial oils are used to function natural fragrances and smells to soaps. They are used for his or her aromatherapeutic powers, and for his or her nutritive rate.

Essential oils are focused compounds extracted from the barks, roots, leaves, seeds, rinds, and flora of plants, each thru a mechanical cold-press method or with the aid of distillation. Essential oils are pure, fragrant and volatile oils, now not much like the base oils which can be an awful lot heavier. They are obviously scented and function the essence of the flowers from which they were derived. They are used to create masses of goods, which includes frame lotions, fragrances, and soaps. They also are used by aromatherapists due to their many health and medicinal advantages.

It's important to get only pure, healing-grade essential oils while the use of them. However, you want to be very cautious while looking for crucial oils, because there are unscrupulous dealers who declare to sell herbal products however dilute their oils with service oils. Some furthermore promote cheaper fragrance oils that have a comparable perfume in location of the actual deal. This is why you need to acquaint your self with who you are seeking out from. Find out how herbal their oil is, in which do they get their product from, and moreover within the event that they have been examined and authorised through the use of a reliable 0.33 celebration.

Frequently, the awareness of the odours that critical oils emit is used to classify them. They can be a top phrase, middle be aware, or base be aware, however, there can be no straight forward class because of the reality many such oils in shape in multiple elegance of notes. It is ordinary practice to encompass oils from the three training of notes, or at least two, while mixing.

Top Notes are sharp, shiny scents which may be most important via manner of the senses. However, they may be fleeting and do now not final extended in advance than fading away. Some of which encompass eucalyptus, peppermint, spearmint, lemongrass, orange, tangerine, lemon, grapefruit, lime, lavender and bergamot.

Middle Notes are less awesome to the senses similar to the pinnacle notes, but they upload greater depth and are longer lasting. They encompass clary sage, clove, cypress, chamomile, juniper berry, rosemary, cinnamon, tea tree, fir needle and geranium.

Base Notes are prolonged-lasting, strong, and heavy. They assist ground and anchor the pinnacle and center notes in a mixture, to cause them to last longer. They encompass cedarwood, patchouli, rose, myrrh, ylang, sandalwood, neroli, helichrysum, frankincense, jasmine, vertices and ginger.

Essential Oil Safety Precautions

Essential oils want to be handled with care, because they're very effective and can reason harm if used indiscriminately. Extra care need to be taken even as the usage of important oils on kids, due to the reality they absorb the ones oils faster into their body; furthermore, it want for use minimally, or now not-at-all, on the aged, on pregnant girls, and on human beings with sure medical situations like diabetes or epilepsy.

Applying vital oils immediately to the pores and skin with out first diluting them with company oils is not suggested. After dilution, constantly conduct a pores and pores and skin patch test to your wrist to make sure you are not allergic to the oil.

All important oils should be averted within the first trimester thru expectant moms. In the second one and third trimester a few critical oils may be used, like lavender, lemongrass, bergamot, lime, lemon, orange, grapefruit, ylang ylang, tea tree, patchouli, litsea and peppermint. Pregnant women and nursing mothers want to avoid clary sage, wintergreen, basil, cinnamon, nutmeg, thyme, clove, cedarwood, rosemary, hyssop and birch.

For children beneath the age of 5 and babies, you could use lavender, chamomile, frankincense, patchouli, cedarwood, cypress, spruce, lemon, bergamot, orange, mandarin, geranium, neroli, juniper berry, tea tree and helichrysum. On the alternative hand, you want to keep away from the usage of eucalyptus, peppermint, wintergreen, rosemary and birch.

Certain vital oils need to be avoided if you are taking prescription treatment or have a certain clinical scenario. Epileptics, as an instance, need to keep away from clary sage, eucalyptus, sweet fennel and rosemary, due to the fact they're stimulating. While mother and father with low blood stress ought to keep away from sage, ylang-ylang and lavender, because of the reality they will be sedatives in nature.

Chapter 4: Cold Process Recipes

CASTILE SOAP

Ingredients:

400g Olive Oil

60g Coconut Oil

60g Shea Butter

138g Sodium Hydroxide (Lye)

300g Distilled Water

10-20g Essential Oil (which incorporates lavender, eucalyptus, or tea tree) - non-obligatory for fragrance

Tools and Equipment:

Safety Gear (gloves, goggles, prolonged sleeves)

Digital Kitchen Scale

Heat-Resistant Containers (for oils and lye answer)

Stick Blender

Soap Mold(s)

Thermometer

Silicone Spatulas

Whisk or Spoon (for mixing lye)

Plastic Wrap or Towel (for insulating the mould)

pH Testing Strips (non-compulsory for trying out)

Instructions:

Safety Note: When handling lye, artwork in an area that is nicely-ventilated and take all vital safety precautions.

1. Prepare: bring together all of your materials and components. And your protecting equipment.

2. Measure Oils and Butters: Weigh the shea butter, coconut oil, and olive oil separately

and location them in warmness-resistant containers.

three. Melt Oils and Butters: Gently melt the coconut oil and shea butter. Olive oil would no longer need to be melted; clearly make certain it is at room temperature.

4. Prepare Lye Solution:

Carefully diploma the distilled water in a warm temperature-resistant region.

Carefully weigh the sodium hydroxide (lye) in a one-of-a-type box.

Stir the lye into the water regularly the usage of a spoon or a whisk. This combination will warmth up and generate fumes, so use warning. Let the lye answer quiet down.

5. Combine Oils and Lye:

Carefully pour the lye solution into the oils once they have both reached a temperature of 100–one hundred ten°F (38–forty 3°C).

Blend the contents with a stick blender till it reaches a mild trace. When the cleaning cleaning soap mixture thickens to the issue in which you could barely make out the blender's faint traces, this is called a hint.

6. Add Essential Oil (Optional):

If you are consisting of critical oil for fragrance, blend it into the cleaning cleaning soap batter at moderate trace. Stir till properly protected.

7. Pour into Mold:

Pour the cleaning soap batter into your cleansing soap mildew(s).

eight. Insulate the Mold:

Cover the mildew with plastic wrap or a towel to insulate it. This allows the soap go through the saponification method.

nine. Curing:

Let the soap take a seat down inside the mould for twenty-4-forty eight hours to harden.

10. Unmold and Cut:

After the preliminary curing period is entire, carefully take the cleaning cleansing cleaning soap from the mold and reduce it into bars.

11. Curing Stage:

The reduce bars have to be placed on a curing rack in a groovy, dry room with splendid airflow. Give the cleaning cleansing soap four-6 weeks to therapy. The cleaning soap hardens and becomes milder at some degree in the curing manner.

12. Test pH (Optional):

If desired, you may test the pH of the cleaning soap after curing the use of pH sorting out strips. Natural Castile cleaning cleaning soap generally has a pH spherical eight-10.

13. Enjoy Your Soap:

Once truely cured, your vegan Castile cleansing cleaning soap is ready to be used and loved!

SHAVING SOAP

Ingredients:

Coconut Oil, 300g

Shea Butter 200g Olive Oil 100g

Castor Oil 100g

50g Cocoa Butter

50g Avocado Oil

135g Sodium Hydroxide (Lye)

300g Distilled Water

1-2 tablespoons Kaolin Clay (for slip and drift)

Essential oils or perfume oils (optionally available)

Natural colorants (optionally available)

Tools:

Safety goggles

Heat-resistant packing containers

Stainless metal or silicone spatulas

Digital kitchen scale

Stick blender

Soap mould

Soap cutter

Thermometer

pH checking out strips (non-compulsory)

Instructions:

Safety Precautions:

Work in a room with properly air flow.

Put on protection device, consisting of gloves and goggles.

To neutralize lye spills, maintain a vinegar or citric acid answer close to hand.

1. Prepare:

Gather all your substances, gear, and protective gear.

Measure your oils and butters the usage of the virtual kitchen scale.

2. Lye Solution:

In a well-ventilated area, regularly add the sodium hydroxide (lye) to the distilled water at the same time as stirring constantly.

Allow the lye manner to chill to around a hundred°F (38°C).

three. Oils and Butters:

In a warm temperature-resistant discipline, melt the avocado oil, shea butter, cocoa butter, and coconut oil. Heat slowly to prevent burning.

Castor oil and olive oil need to be brought to the melted aggregate.

4. Combine Lye and Oils:

Make that the temperature of the lye answer and oil mixture are each close to one hundred°F (38°C).

Pour the lye solution into the oils frequently as you whisk with a spatula.

five. Emulsify:

Use a stick blender to mixture the components up till a mild trace is finished. This suggests that the aggregate has slightly thickened.

6. Add Kaolin Clay and Essential Oils:

For slip and float, blend in 1-2 teaspoons of kaolin clay to the cleaning cleaning soap batter.

Add perfume or important oils for a nice fragrance, if desired. Start with 20 to 30 drops and then titrate as favored.

7. Pour into Mold:

Fill your cleansing soap mold with the cleaning soap batter.

eight. Tap and Settle:

To cast off air bubbles and ensure the cleaning soap falls flippantly, gently tap the mildew towards a countertop.

nine. Insulate and Cure:

Use a stick blender to aggregate the additives up until a slight trace is carried out.

Give the cleaning soap 24-48 hours to remedy within the mold.

10. Unmold and Cut:

After the preliminary curing duration, take the cleaning cleaning soap out of the mold and use a cleaning soap cutter to reduce it into the popular shapes.

eleven. Cure Further:

On a curing rack in a well-ventilated vicinity, installation the lessen cleaning cleansing soap bars.

For the soap to properly saponify and gain its maximum excellent, deliver it four-6 weeks to remedy.

12. Test and Enjoy:

After the curing length, you can check the pH the usage of attempting out strips to make certain the cleaning cleansing cleaning soap is slight.

Your herbal vegan shaving cleaning cleansing cleaning soap is now equipped for use. Enjoy a highly-priced and pores and pores and pores and skin-exceptional shaving revel in!

SHAMPOO SOAP

Ingredients:

300g Coconut Oil

200g Olive Oil

100g Castor Oil

100g Shea Butter

90g Sodium Hydroxide (Lye)

200ml Distilled Water

1 tablespoon of Nettle Powder (herbal hair care)

15-20g Essential Oils (which includes Lavender, Rosemary, or Tea Tree)

Tools:

Safety goggles

Gloves

Digital kitchen scale

Heat-stable bins (stainless-steel or heat-resistant plastic)

Stick blender

Soap mould

Thermometer

Stirring utensils

Protective clothing

Instructions:

1. Safety Precautions: Put on safety goggles and gloves, and paintings in a properly-ventilated area.

2. Measure Ingredients: Weigh each oil and the lye appropriately the usage of a digital kitchen scale.

3. Prepare Lye Solution:

To the distilled water, upload the lye. DON'T mix water with lye.

Gently stir the aggregate till all the lye has been dissolved. The mixture becomes very hot. Allow it to sit down lower back to around 100°F (38°C).

4. Melt Oils and Butters:

Castor oil, coconut oil, olive oil, and shea butter have to all be melted in a warmness-steady vessel. Use a hob or microwave on low warm temperature.

The oils want to be allowed to loosen up to approximately a hundred°F (38°C).

5. Prepare Soap Mold:

Use a silicone mould or line your cleaning cleansing cleaning soap mould with parchment paper.

6. Combine Lye Solution and Oils:

Use a silicone mould or line your cleaning soap mildew with parchment paper.

7. Blend and Reach Trace:

Till you reach hint, integrate the oils and lye the usage of a stick blender. The aggregate has the feel of thin custard when it has reached the trace stage.

8. Add Nettle Powder and Essential Oils:

Add nettle powder for herbal hair care blessings and crucial oils for fragrance. Mix very well.

9. Pour into Mold:

Pour the cleaning cleaning soap combination into the organized mould.

10. Insulate and Cure:

Place the mould in a heat, quiet area and cowl it with a bit of cardboard or a towel. This aids in accelerating the saponification system.

Give the cleaning soap 24-48 hours to relaxation in the mold.

11. Unmold and Cut:

Once the cleansing cleaning soap has set, dispose of it from the mildew and decrease it into bars the usage of a pointy knife.

12. Curing:

On a curing rack in a cool, dry, and nicely-ventilated location, installation the reduce cleaning cleaning soap bars.

Give the soap bars 4-6 weeks to treatment. The greater moisture will evaporate at some stage in this era, making the cleaning cleaning soap softer and less assailable.

13. Enjoy:
After the curing duration, your natural vegan shampoo soap is ready to use!

LAUNDRY SOAP

Ingredients:

Coconut Oil, 350g

Olive Oil, 150g

Sunflower Oil, 100g

300g of distilled water, 135g of sodium hydroxide (lye), and 100g of castor oil

30-40g Essential Oil (Lavender, Tea Tree, or Lemon)

1 tablespoon Sodium Bicarbonate (Baking Soda) (optionally to be had, for extra cleaning energy)

Tools:

Safety tools (gloves, goggles, lengthy sleeves)

Digital scale

Heat-resistant boxes

Stick blender

Soap mold

Plastic wrap or parchment paper

Instructions:

1. Safety first: Protect yourself from lye via the use of protecting system and taking the vital protection measures.

2. Oil Measurement: In separate warmness-resistant packing containers, weigh the castor oil, coconut oil, olive oil, and sunflower oil.

three. Measure the lye (sodium hydroxide) and water one after the alternative, being careful to accomplish that.

four. Lye solution combined: Stirring constantly, often add the lye to the water. Do this in a room with authentic air float. Heat and scents may be launched from the mixture. The lye solution want to be allowed to chill to approximately one hundred°F (38°C).

5. Melt Oils: Warm coconut oil until in reality melted over a low flame. Let it cool to approximately 100°F (38°C).

6. Combine Lye and Oils: When the lye answer and the oils have both warmed to spherical one hundred°F (38°C), slowly pour the lye answer into the melting oils. Use a stick blender to mixture until you achieve a mild hint, that is need to a skinny custard.

7. Add the chosen important oil for perfume and the sodium bicarbonate (baking soda) at your discretion for added cleaning electricity. Mix till in reality blended.

8. Pour into Mold: Fill your cleaning cleaning soap mildew with the cleaning soap batter. To eliminate any air bubbles, gently faucet the mildew on a flat floor.

9. Insulate and remedy: Wrap the mildew in plastic wrap or parchment paper to insulate it. Allow the soap to harden up inside the mildew for twenty-four to 48 hours.

10. Unmold and Cut: After the cleaning soap has dried, cautiously take it out of the mildew and use a knife or cleansing soap cutter to reduce it into bars.

11. Place the reduce bars on a drying rack and hold them someplace cold and dry to treatment. Allow them to heal for 4-6 weeks. This permits more water to break out, making the cleansing soap extra hard and gentler as a quit result.

12. Test and Use: After the curing duration, check a small piece of soap on your laundry to make certain it cleans efficiently and might no longer depart any residue. If glad, you may start the usage of your herbal vegan laundry cleaning cleaning soap!

TEA TREE CHARCOAL SOAP

Ingredients:

300g coconut oil

150g olive oil

150g shea butter

50g castor oil

140g distilled water

65g sodium hydroxide (lye)

10g tea tree essential oil

1 tablespoon activated charcoal powder

Tools:

Safety device (gloves, goggles, prolonged sleeves)

Digital kitchen scale

Heat-resistant boxes

Stick blender

Soap mold

Thermometer

Mixing spoons

Measuring spoons

Plastic wrap or fabric

Plastic wrap or lid for the mould

Instructions:

Safety Precautions:

1. Wear the best safety gadget and paintings in a region this is nicely-ventilated (gloves, goggles, lengthy sleeves).

Prepare:

2. Using a digital kitchen scale, exactly diploma each issue.

three. Line your cleaning soap mould with plastic wrap or a piece of material to put together it. Leave it on my own.

Mix Lye Solution:

four. Carefully mixture the distilled water with the sodium hydroxide (lye) in a properly-ventilated room. Stir until the whole thing is dissolved. This solution heats up brief, so use caution. Set apart for cooling.

Melt Oils:

5. In a warmness-resistant container, soften castor oil, shea butter, coconut oil, and olive oil. Use a double boiler or the microwave for restricted periods to keep away from overheating. The oils want to be allowed to loosen up to about 100°F (38°C).

Prepare Soap Batter:

6. The lye answer and oils need to each be at or near 100°F (38°C).

7. Gradually add the lye method to the oils. When the aggregate has a slight trace and resembles skinny custard, combine with a stick blender.

Add Essential Oil and Charcoal:

8. The cleaning cleaning soap batter must moreover incorporate powdered activated charcoal and tea tree important oil. Mix the whole thing very well until it's miles distributed lightly.

Pour into Mold:

nine. Fill the prepared cleaning soap mold with the cleansing soap batter.

Smooth and Cover:

10. To eliminate air bubbles, gently tap the mildew on a floor.

eleven. To even out the cleaning cleaning soap's top, use a spoon or spatula.

12. Wrap the mould in plastic wrap or a lid to insulate it and preserve it undisturbed.

Curing:

thirteen. Give the cleaning soap 24 to 48 hours to enterprise and saponify in the mildew.

14. Carefully put off the cleaning soap from the mildew as fast as the preliminary curing method is complete, then reduce it into bars.

Cure Further:

Put the reduce bars on a curing rack and place them far from direct sunlight in a nicely-ventilated room. Give them 4 to six weeks to heal. This curing duration aids within the entire hardening of the cleansing cleaning soap and makes it gentler for use.

Enjoy:

Once the curing period is entire, your vegan tea tree charcoal soap is prepared to apply or gift.

Chapter 5: Blue Lavender Soap

Ingredients:

Coconut Oil: 300g

Olive Oil: 300g

Shea Butter: 100g

Castor Oil: 50g

Sodium Hydroxide (Lye): 77g

Distilled Water: 150g

Lavender Essential Oil: 15g

Blue Mica Powder (Skin-Safe): half of of tsp

Dried Lavender Buds (optionally available): 1 tbsp

Tools:

Safety goggles and gloves

Digital kitchen scale

Heat-resistant containers

Stick blender

Soap mould

Mixing spoons

Thermometer

Plastic wrap or material for insulating

Instructions:

1. Safety First: Wear protection goggles and gloves whilst running with lye. Work in a nicely-ventilated vicinity.

2. Measure Ingredients: Shea butter, castor oil, coconut oil, and olive oil must all be weighed one after the alternative.

3. Lye Solution:

Carefully add the lye to distilled water (now not the opportunity manner around) in a warm temperature-resistant location. Shake till dissolved. Heat and scents might be launched via way of the combination.

Let the lye answer cool to approximately 110°F (forty three°C).

four. Melt Oils: Shea butter, coconut oil, and olive oil should all be melted collectively. Gently warm temperature within the microwave or at the hob till without a doubt melted. Allow it to relax to approximately 110 °F (forty 3 °C).

5. Prepare Soap Mold: Cover the cleaning cleaning soap mould with fabric or plastic wrap. This step might not be important if using silicone moulds.

6. Mixing: Pouring the lye answer into the melted oils lightly at the same time as stirring with a spoon or stick blender.

7. Blend to Trace: Mix the oils and lye answer with a stick blender till it reaches hint. Trace takes region whilst the aggregate turns into thick enough to resemble pudding.

8. Add Essential Oil and Colorant:

Add lavender crucial oil to the soap batter. Stir to consist of.

Mix the blue mica powder with a small quantity of provider oil or a portion of the cleaning cleansing cleaning soap batter to create a clean mixture. Add this coloured aggregate to the cleaning cleaning soap batter and mix till flippantly coloured.

9. Pour into Mold: Pour the coloured cleansing cleaning soap batter into the organized mould.

10. Texture (Optional): If preferred, sprinkle dried lavender buds on pinnacle of the cleansing cleansing cleaning soap to characteristic texture and visible interest.

11. Insulation: Cover the mildew with plastic wrap or a cloth to insulate. This allows the saponification machine for the cleaning cleansing soap.

12. Curing: For the cleansing cleaning soap to corporation up, leave it inside the mildew for twenty-4 to 48 hours. The cleaning cleaning soap must then be lightly taken out of the mould and reduce into bars.

thirteen. Curing Period: Place the reduce bars in a nicely-ventilated location or on a curing rack. Cure the cleansing soap for four to six weeks to allow it to completely saponify and become milder on the pores and skin.

14. Enjoy: Once cured, your vegan blue lavender cleansing cleaning soap is prepared to apply! Store any more cleaning soap in a fab, dry region.

GREEN TEA & ALOE SOAP

300g Coconut Oil

200g Olive Oil

150g Shea Butter

100g Castor Oil

85g Sodium Hydroxide (Lye)

200g Distilled Water

1 Green Tea Bag

1 tablespoon Green Tea Powder

2 tablespoons Aloe Vera Gel

Essential Oils (non-obligatory, for fragrance)

Soap Mold

Safety Gear (gloves, goggles)

Mixing Bowls

Stick Blender

Thermometer

Instructions:

1. Safety First: Put on your safety system, along with gloves and goggles, in a well-ventilated location.

2. Brew Green Tea:

Steep the green tea bag in a small amount of distilled water. Let it cool and set apart.

3. Prepare Ingredients:

Weigh the olive oil, castor oil, shea butter, and coconut oil. The strong oils (coconut oil and shea butter) need to be slowly melted over slight warmth.

4. Measure Lye and Water:

Carefully degree the lye the use of a digital scale. Measure the final distilled water one at a time.

five. Mix Lye Solution:

Gently mixture the water as you frequently upload the lye. Let the lye answer relax.

6. Prepare Green Tea Infusion:

Remove the tea bag from the brewed inexperienced tea. Add the green tea powder to the tea and blend nicely.

7. Combine Oils and Lye:

Pour the lye answer into the oils cautiously once they have every reached a temperature of round 100°F (38°C). Mix everything with a stick blender till hint is reached.

eight. Add Green Tea and Aloe:

Add the inexperienced tea infusion and aloe vera gel to the soap combination. Blend till properly included.

9. Scent and Mold:

If the usage of critical oils, upload them to the cleansing soap aggregate and mix in short. Pour the soap combination into your soap mildew.

10. Tap and Insulate:

To allow air bubbles out, lightly tap the mould on a surface. To insulate the mould, cover it with a chunk of cardboard after which wrap it in a towel or blanket.

11. Cure:

Leave the cleaning soap in the mould for twenty-four-48 hours. Afterward, unmold and reduce the cleansing cleaning soap into bars.

12. Curing Period:

In a fab, dry place, set up the reduce soap bars on a curing rack. Give them 4-6 weeks to heal. This lets in the cleaning cleaning soap to well harden and saponify.

13. Enjoy:

Once completely cured, your inexperienced tea and aloe vera vegan cleaning soap is ready to apply. Enjoy the pores and skin-nourishing benefits with every use!

Hot-Processed Soap Recipes

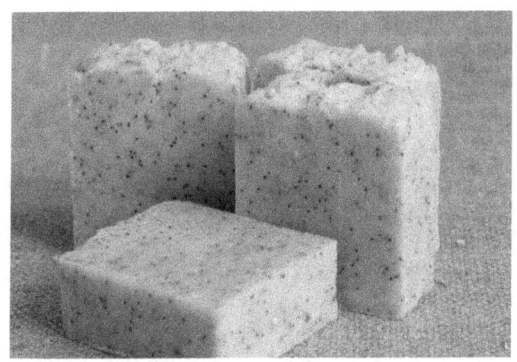

Cold and warm approach soapmaking are comparable procedures, with the identical strategies, dosages, and component necessities. The heat machine starts offevolved with the cleansing soap batter starting to hint, that is cooked to rush up the saponification technique. This step lets in for the addition of colourants, fragrances, and one of a kind additions to create odours so that you can linger longer. The cleansing soap can be used immediately, but it is encouraged to permit it sit for 24 hours to consistent with week to permit water to evaporate and harden.

Hot way soaps have a country look and are more tough to enhance with complicated strategies because of their thicker texture. However, allowing the cleaning soap to remedy for 2-4 weeks can result in a more exquisite cleaning soap that lasts longer. Colorants and different additives may be added all through the lye answer aggregate with base oils or after saponification even as the cleaning cleaning soap reaches gel section. To advantage a extra fluid cleansing cleaning cleaning soap batter, additives like yogurt, sodium lactate, and/or sugars like maple syrup, honey, and agave may be delivered to help loosen it.

HOT PROCESS RECIPES

NETTLE LEAF FLORAL SOAP

Ingredients:

250g coconut oil

200g olive oil

150g shea butter

50g castor oil

120g sodium hydroxide (lye)

260g distilled water

2 tablespoons dried nettle leaves

1 teaspoon lavender critical oil

1 teaspoon geranium essential oil

Dried flower petals (which includes rose petals, calendula petals, or lavender buds) for adornment

Tools:

Heat-secure boxes (for measuring and mixing)

Stick blender

Stainless metal or warmth-resistant plastic spatula

Safety goggles and gloves

Soap mould

Crockpot or sluggish cooker

Digital kitchen scale

Immersion blender

Thermometer

Plastic wrap or parchment paper

Instructions:

Preparation:

1. Safety First: Wear safety goggles and gloves at some diploma in the soapmaking manner. Work in a nicely-ventilated location.

Soap Making:

1. Measure Ingredients:

Weigh the castor oil, shea butter, olive oil, and coconut oil separately in warmth-stable boxes. Measure the distilled water and sodium hydroxide as nicely.

2. Mix Lye Solution:

Add the sodium hydroxide slowly to the distilled water and stir till it dissolves in a well-ventilated surroundings. Allow the lye technique to chill to spherical one hundred ten°F (forty three°C).

three. Melt Oils:

Combine the castor oil, shea butter, coconut oil, and olive oil in a warmth-strong container. Use the burner or microwave to slowly melt the oils.

four. Infuse Nettle Leaves:

Place the dried nettle leaves in a warmth-stable problem. Infuse the nettle leaves with a hint amount of heated oil with the aid of way of pouring it over them. Allow the leaves to steep at the same time as the oils lighten up.

5. Combine Lye and Oils:

Once the oils and lye solution are each round 110°F (40 3°C), cautiously pour the lye solution into the melted oils, stirring lightly.

6. Immersion Blend:

Using an immersion blender, very well integrate the aggregate until it has a slight hint. This is while the mixture thickens slightly.

7. Cooking (Hot Process):

Transfer the cleansing soap batter to a crockpot or sluggish cooker set on low warmth. Cook the cleaning soap batter while stirring sometimes. The cleaning cleaning soap will undergo diverse stages and become translucent and remarkable.

eight. Check for Doneness:

Test the cleansing cleansing soap's readiness by way of manner of acting a zap check. If there can be no zap (tingling sensation) on your tongue whilst you contact a small amount of soap, it is ready.

9. Add Essential Oils:

Once the cleaning cleaning soap has reached the favored consistency and is without a doubt cooked, turn off the warm temperature. Add the lavender and geranium essential oils and stir nicely to include.

Molding and Curing:

1. Add Decorations:

Line your cleaning soap mildew with parchment paper or plastic wrap. Press dried flower petals onto the lowest of the mildew for decorative accents.

2. Pour and Shape:

Carefully transfer the new cleansing cleaning cleaning soap aggregate into the mildew, spreading It calmly. Gently faucet the mould to remove air bubbles.

3. Cool and Cut:

Allow the cleaning soap to relax and solidify within the mildew for some hours. When the cleaning cleaning soap has cooled, take it out of the mold and decrease it into bars.

four. Curing:

Place the reduce soap bars on a drying rack in a groovy, dry place. Give them one to 2 weeks to heal. Hot device soap treatment options greater brief than bloodless gadget cleaning cleaning soap.

Final Touches:

Labeling and Storage:

Once the cleaning cleansing soap bars are in fact cured, you can label them with their components and date of advent. Store them in a dry region a long way from direct sunlight hours.

SEAWEED ORANGE SOAP

Ingredients:

250g coconut oil

200g olive oil

100g shea butter

50g castor oil

70g sodium hydroxide (lye)

160g distilled water

2 tablespoons dried seaweed (finely floor)

15-20 drops orange essential oil

1 teaspoon spirulina powder (for color, non-compulsory)

Tools:

Heat-resistant glass or chrome steel packing containers

Stick blender

Digital kitchen scale

Protective device (gloves, goggles, lengthy sleeves)

Silicone mold

Stainless metal or warmth-resistant spatula

Crockpot or slow cooker

pH checking out strips (non-compulsory)

Soap cutter

Instructions:

1. Prepare:

Wear protecting equipment to ensure safety.

Measure and put together all factors and system.

2. Make Lye Solution:

In a well-ventilated region, cautiously upload sodium hydroxide to distilled water. Stir till absolutely dissolved. Allow the lye approach to chill.

three. Melt Oils:

In the crockpot, melt coconut oil, olive oil, shea butter, and castor oil on low warmth.

four. Combine Lye Solution and Oils:

Pour the lye answer into the melted oils regularly whilst the lye solution and the oils have every cooled to approximately one hundred ten°F (forty three°C). Stir the usage of a warmth-resistant or stainless steel spatula.

5. Blend and Cook:

Blend the combination with a stick blender until it reaches trace (the issue at which it thickens to a pudding-like consistency).

Cover the crockpot and prepare dinner dinner the cleaning soap on low warmness. Stir every now and then to prevent sizzling.

6. Check Soap Consistency:

After approximately 30-forty mins, the cleaning cleaning soap should have cooked sufficiently and transformed proper proper right into a translucent and homogeneous texture.

7. Add Seaweed and Color:

Add the finely floor dried seaweed and spirulina powder (if using) to the cleansing soap combination. Stir well to distribute frivolously.

eight. Scent with Orange Essential Oil:

Add 15-20 drops of orange important oil to the cleansing cleaning cleaning soap mixture. Stir to contain the heady scent.

nine. Test pH (Optional):

If desired, you can test the pH of the cleaning soap the usage of pH attempting out strips. The pH of warm technique cleaning cleaning soap generally ranges from 8 to 10.

10. Mold the Soap:

Spoon the cleaning cleaning cleaning soap combination right into a silicone mould, ensuring it's far gently allotted.

eleven. Let the Soap Cool and Set:

Allow the cleaning cleansing soap to chill and harden in the mildew for some hours.

12. Unmold and Cut:

Once the cleaning cleaning soap has completely cooled and hardened, lightly unmold it from the silicone mildew.

thirteen. Cure:

Hot approach soap may be used quite speedy after cooling but allowing it to remedy for some weeks will bring about a milder and longer-lasting bar.

HONEY, LEMON & OATMEAL SOAP

Ingredients:

300g Coconut Oil

200g Olive Oil

100g Shea Butter

50g Castor Oil

140g Sodium Hydroxide (Lye)

320g Distilled Water

three tbsp Oatmeal

2 tbsp Lemon Zest (dried or smooth)

1 tbsp Lemon Essential Oil

1 tbsp Honey (for vegan possibility, use agave or maple syrup)

Optional: Yellow herbal colorant (like turmeric), for colour

Tools:

Heat-resistant bins

Stainless metal pot for blending oils

Mixing spoons (chrome steel or silicone)

Digital kitchen scale

Stick blender

Thermometer

Soap mold

Safety tools (gloves, goggles, lengthy sleeves)

Parchment paper (to line mildew)

Instructions:

1. Safety First:

Put on protection equipment: gloves, goggles, and lengthy sleeves.

Work in a nicely-ventilated region.

2. Measure Ingredients:

Measure all additives using a digital kitchen scale. Keep sodium hydroxide (lye) lessen loose unique substances.

3. Prepare Lemon Zest and Oatmeal:

Grate lemon zest and set aside.

Oatmeal should be finely ground the use of a blender or meals processor. This permits to save you a tough texture in the cleansing soap.

4. Mix Lye Solution:

In a nicely-ventilated vicinity, cautiously upload lye to distilled water (not the alternative way round) on the same time as stirring. Allow the lye method to kick back to round a hundred°F (38°C).

five. Combine Oils:

Combine coconut oil, olive oil, shea butter, and castor oil in a chrome steel kettle. Heat the oils on low warmth till completely melted.

6. Mix Lye Solution and Oils:

Check the temperatures of the lye solution and oils. Both have to be spherical a hundred°F (38°C).

Slowly pour the lye answer into the oils at the same time as stirring with a spoon or stick blender.

7. Blend to Trace:

Blend the aggregate using a stick blender until it reaches "hint," which is a thickened consistency similar to custard.

eight. Add Lemon Zest, Oatmeal, and Colorant:

Add lemon zest, floor oatmeal, and a small amount of yellow natural colorant if desired. Mix nicely.

nine. Cook the Soap:

On low warm temperature, preserve to simmer the cleaning soap mixture, stirring from time to time to save you sticking. It will undergo severa degrees, turning into translucent and jelly-like.

10. Add Lemon Essential Oil and Honey:

Once the cleansing cleansing soap reaches a mashed potato-like consistency, flip off the warmth.

Stir in lemon crucial oil and honey (or vegan opportunity). Mix thoroughly.

eleven. Mold the Soap:

Line the cleaning cleansing soap mold with parchment paper.

Pour the cleansing cleaning soap mixture into the mildew and press it down calmly.

12. Cool and Cut:

Spend many hours or the complete night time letting the cleaning soap cool and set inside the mildew.

After the cleansing soap has virtually cooled, carefully take it from the mould and decrease it into bars.

thirteen. Cure and Enjoy:

The reduce bars want to be positioned on a curing rack and permit to treatment for 4-6 weeks. The cleansing cleaning soap receives softer and gentler over this era.

After curing, your herbal vegan honey, lemon & oatmeal cleaning cleaning soap is ready to use and revel in!

PUMPKIN TURMERIC SOAP

Ingredients:

2 liters of coconut oil

Olive oil, hundred grams

Shea butter 100 grams

zero.5 g of castor oil

sodium hydroxide, one hundred twenty 5 grams (lye)

250 grams of herbal water

2 teaspoons of pureed pumpkin (unsweetened)

one teaspoon of turmeric powder

ten to fifteen drops of vital oil (together with candy orange or cinnamon)

Decorative dried calendula petals are non-obligatory.

Tools:

Safety device (gloves, goggles)

Heat-safe packing containers

Stainless metal or warmth-resistant plastic utensils

Stick blender

Soap mold

Crockpot or slow cooker

Digital kitchen scale

pH finding out strips (for non-compulsory pH checking out)

Instructions:

1. Safety First:

Put for your safety equipment, inclusive of gloves and goggles, to defend yourself on the same time as dealing with lye.

2. Measure Ingredients:

Weigh all oils (coconut, olive, shea butter, castor) one after the other using the virtual kitchen scale.

3. Prepare Lye Solution:

Prepare the lye answer by using manner of carefully blending the distilled water with sodium hydroxide (lye) in a nicely-ventilated area. Stirring is needed to honestly dissolve the lye. Let the answer cool to round a hundred°F (38°C).

four. Prepare Pumpkin Puree:

In a small bowl, mix the pumpkin puree and turmeric powder till nicely mixed. Set apart.

5. Combine Oils:

In the gradual cooker, blend the castor oil, shea butter, coconut oil, and olive oil. Set the crockpot's warmth to low.

6. Melt Oils:

Allow the oils to melt and blend together within the crockpot. Aim for a temperature of round 100 twenty°F (40 nine°C).

7. Add Lye Solution:

Pour the lye solution into the melted oils with warning. Stir lightly using a warmness-resistant plastic or stainless-steel utensil.

eight. Blend the Soap Mixture:

The cleansing cleansing cleaning soap aggregate have to be blended with a stick blender until it reaches a faint trace. The aggregate have to resemble thin pudding.

nine. Cook the Soap:

Continue cooking the cleaning soap combination inside the crockpot on low warmth. Stir sometimes to save you sticking.

10. Add Pumpkin Turmeric Mixture:

When the cleaning soap mixture is cooked (reaches a gel-like consistency and turns translucent), upload the pumpkin turmeric mixture and vital oil. Stir well to truly encompass.

eleven. Check for "Vaseline Stage":

To test if the cleaning cleaning soap is prepared, carry out the "vaseline diploma" check. Take a small quantity of cleaning soap and rub it amongst your palms. If it feels easy and "vaseline-like," the soap is prepared.

12. Mold the Soap:

Turn off the crockpot and carefully switch the cleansing soap mixture into the cleaning soap mildew. If preferred, press dried calendula petals onto the pinnacle for decoration.

thirteen. Cool and Cut:

Spend many hours or the entire night time time letting the cleaning soap cool and set within the mildew. Carefully remove the cleaning soap from the mold once it has surely cooled and set, then slice it into bars.

14. Curing:

In a cool, dry region, set up the lessen cleansing soap bars on a curing rack. Allow them to treatment for 4 to 6 weeks. The cleansing cleaning cleaning soap will keep to harden inside the route of this era, and the pH degree will stabilise.

15. Enjoy:

Your vegan pumpkin turmeric cleaning soap is ready for use after it has dried. Take benefit of the pores and skin-pleasant traits of this nourishing cleaning cleaning soap's lovely aroma.

CUCUMBER & ALOE VERA SOAP

Ingredients:

300g Coconut Oil

200g Olive Oil

100g Sunflower Oil

100g Shea Butter

110g Sodium Hydroxide (Lye)

250g Distilled Water

1 medium Cucumber (peeled and pureed)

50g Aloe Vera Gel

15g Cucumber Seed Oil

15g Castor Oil

15g Cucumber Fragrance Oil (or essential oil of preference)

1 teaspoon Green Spirulina Powder (for colour, optionally available)

1 teaspoon White Kaolin Clay (for texture, non-obligatory)

Tools:

Digital kitchen scale

Heat-resistant bins

Mixing utensils (stainless steel or warmness-resistant)

Stick blender

Soap mould

Safety equipment (gloves, goggles, long sleeves)

Instructions:

Safety Note: The caustic chemical lye is used within the production of cleansing cleansing soap. Wear the proper protection device and paintings in a nicely-ventilated location constantly.

1. Prepare Ingredients

Measure all oils (coconut, olive, sunflower, shea butter, cucumber seed oil, and castor oil) and vicinity them in a warm temperature-resistant box.

Measure distilled water and lye one at a time in super bins.

2. Mix Lye Solution

Carefully whisk lye into distilled water earlier than adding extra. As you keep, permit this combination cool as it will warmness up.

3. Heat Oils

Heat the measured oils in a double boiler until they're certainly melted.

four. Combine Lye Solution and Oils

Pour the lye answer into the oils slowly at the equal time as swirling them lightly as quickly because the oils and lye solution have each cooled to approximately a hundred-one hundred ten°F (38-forty three°C).

five. Blend and Reach Trace

The oils and lye solution have to be blended with a stick blender until they have got a slight hint. When the aggregate reaches the hint degree, dripped strains are regardless of the fact that discernible at the floor.

6. Add Cucumber Puree

Add the peeled and pureed cucumber to the cleansing cleaning cleaning soap combination. Blend it in using the stick blender till nicely included.

7. Cook the Soap

Transfer the cleaning cleaning soap combination to a warm temperature-resistant pot or slow cooker. Cover and put together dinner dinner on low warmth for about 1-2 hours, stirring now and again.

eight. Check the Soap's Consistency

The soap will undergo stages of "gel segment." It will begin searching translucent after which go back to an opaque look. When the soap is definitely cooked, it ought to resemble mashed potatoes and feature a smooth look.

nine. Add Aloe Vera Gel and Fragrance

Once the cleansing cleaning soap is genuinely cooked, flip off the warmth. Add the aloe vera gel, cucumber fragrance oil, and any non-compulsory colorants (like spirulina powder) and texture enhancers (like white kaolin clay). Mix properly.

10. Mold the Soap

Quickly transfer the cleansing cleaning soap mixture into your cleaning soap mildew. Press it down evenly.

eleven. Cut and Cure

After 24-forty eight hours, the cleansing cleaning soap have to be organisation sufficient to unmold and reduce into bars.

The lessen bars want to be stored in a fab, dry region to treatment for 4-6 weeks. The cleaning soap will solidify and any greater water will evaporate within the route of this period, growing a softer and longer-lasting bar.

CILANTRO SOAP

Ingredients:

300g coconut oil

200g olive oil

150g shea butter

100g avocado oil

75g castor oil

130g distilled water

60g sodium hydroxide (lye)

15g sparkling cilantro leaves (finely chopped)

15g cilantro essential oil

Green oxide or spinach powder (herbal colorant)

Tools:

Digital kitchen scale

Heat-steady containers

Soap mold

Immersion blender

Silicone spatulas

Safety goggles and gloves

Protective apparel

Stick blender

Stainless steel or tooth pot

Instructions:

Safety Precautions:

1. Ensure you're carrying defensive system – safety goggles, gloves, and appropriate clothing.

2. Work in a properly-ventilated location.

three. Always add lye to water, in no manner the opposite manner spherical.

Soap Making Process:

1. Measure Oils: Weigh the castor oil, avocado oil, shea butter, coconut oil, and

olive oil. In a warmness-resistant container, integrate them.

2. Melt Oils: Gently warm temperature the oils until actually melted, the usage of a double boiler or microwave.

three. Prepare Lye Solution: In a separate problem, carefully diploma distilled water. Slowly upload sodium hydroxide (lye) to the water on the same time as stirring. Allow the lye method to chill.

4. Mix Oils and Lye Solution: Once every the oils and the lye solution have heated to a temperature of round 110-one hundred twenty°F (forty three-40 9°C), carefully pour the lye solution into the oils. The factors must be blended with an immersion blender till it reaches hint (a pudding-like consistency).

five. Cook the Soap: Put the cleaning soap combination in an enamel or stainless-steel pot. Cook the cleansing cleaning soap within the pot over low warmness, stirring now and again. As the cleansing cleaning soap cooks, it'll undergo severa levels and turn out to be translucent and slightly gel-like.

6. Add Cilantro: When the cleansing cleaning soap is completely cooked and has a mashed potato-like consistency, turn off the warmth. Add the chopped cilantro leaves and cilantro important oil to the combination. Mix well.

7. Color the Soap: Add a pinch of inexperienced oxide or spinach powder to reap a natural inexperienced color. Mix well till the coloration is dispersed calmly.

8. Transfer to Mold: Quickly switch the cleaning soap combination into your cleansing cleaning soap mold, using a silicone spatula to flatten the top.

9. Cool and Cure: Allow the cleaning soap to relax and harden in the mildew for approximately 24 hours.

10. Cut and Cure: Once the cleansing cleaning soap has absolutely cooled, remove it from the mildew with care in advance than reducing it into bars. To allow greater

moisture to interrupt out and the cleaning soap to grow to be gentler and remaining longer, area the bars on a drying rack and allow them to remedy for about 3–4 weeks.

11. Enjoy: Your Vegan Cilantro Soap is ready to use once the curing approach is finished. A revitalizing cleansing sensation is probably supplied through the energizing oils and the aromatic cilantro.

Chapter 6: Shea Butter Vanilla Coffee Soap

Ingredients:

Coconut oil, 200g

Shea butter, 150g

Olive oil, 100g

Castor oil, 50g

70g sodium hydroxide (lye)

180g brewed coffee (room temperature)

20g vanilla crucial oil (or perfume oil)

2 tablespoons finely ground coffee

1 teaspoon cocoa powder (for color, non-obligatory)

Tools:

Safety goggles and gloves

Digital kitchen scale

Heat-resistant boxes

Stick blender

Stainless metallic or warm temperature-resistant plastic blending utensils

Crockpot or slow cooker

Soap mildew

Parchment paper or plastic wrap (for lining the mildew)

Instructions:

Safety Precautions:

1. Safety Gear: Wear safety goggles and gloves to shield your eyes and pores and pores and skin whilst walking with lye.

Preparing:

2. Measure Ingredients: Weigh all of the oils (coconut, shea, olive, castor) one after the other of their respective bins.

3. Brew Coffee: Brew the coffee and allow it cool to room temperature. This can be your liquid element.

four. Prepare Mold: For later elimination, line the cleansing cleaning soap mould with parchment paper or plastic wrap.

Lye Solution:

5. Mix Lye: Carefully stir sodium hydroxide (lye) into the brewed coffee in a nicely-ventilated room. Gently stir till the whole thing is dissolved. The concoction will warmth up. Set aside for cooling.

Oil Mixture:

6. Melt Oils: Melt the olive oil, coconut oil, and shea butter over low warmth in a warmth-resistant bowl or in the sluggish cooker's base.

7. Combine Oils: Once the oils are melted, eliminate from heat and add castor oil. The aggregate should be warmth, not heat.

Soap Making Process:

eight. Add Lye to Oils: Pour the lye solution into the heating oils regularly and lightly.

Blend the contents with a stick blender till it reaches a mild trace.

nine. Cook Soap: Transfer the mixture into the gradual cooker set on low warmth. Cook the cleansing cleaning cleaning soap, stirring on occasion, until it is going through a gel phase (turns into translucent and heated throughout).

10. Check for Doneness: The cleansing cleaning soap is prepared when it resembles mashed potatoes, and you can see "Vaseline-like" streaks. This can take spherical 1-2 hours.

11. Add Vanilla and Coffee: Turn off the warm temperature. Stir in vanilla crucial oil (or perfume oil), finely floor espresso, and cocoa powder (if the usage of) to offer the cleansing cleaning soap a rich shade and espresso scent.

Molding and Curing:

12. Transfer to Mold: Spoon the cleaning cleaning soap mixture cautiously into the

organized mold. Use a spatula or the decrease returned of a spoon to level the top.

thirteen. Cool and Set: Let the cleaning soap cool and harden inside the mould for as a minimum 24 hours.

14. Unmold and Cut: Once fully cooled and set, dispose of the cleansing cleaning cleaning soap from the mould. Cut it into bars of your selected length.

15. Curing: The lessen bars ought to be dried for four-6 weeks on a drying rack in a properly-ventilated environment. This lets in extra water to evaporate, making the cleansing cleansing soap more difficult and additional durable.

sixteen. Enjoy: Once cured, your vegan shea butter vanilla coffee cleaning cleansing soap is ready to be used! The shea butter and oils provide extraordinary moisture for your skin, at the identical time because the coffee grounds offer moderate exfoliation.

COCONUT MILK WITH SHEA BUTTER SOAP

Ingredients:

Coconut oil, 100 seventy grams

Olive oil, a hundred and seventy grams

Shea butter 80 five grams

Sunflower oil, 80 five grams

a hundred and fifty grams of water, distilled

sodium hydroxide, 73 grams (lye)

a hundred grams of coconut milk in a can (whole-fat, unsweetened)

10 grams of herbal oil (inclusive of lavender, tea tree, or citrus)

Natural dyes (clays, spirulina) and dried plants for redecorating are non-obligatory.

Tools:

Safety gadget (gloves, goggles)

Stainless steel or warm temperature-resistant plastic packing containers

Digital kitchen scale

Stick blender

Stainless metal or warmth-resistant plastic spoon

Soap mould

Parchment paper or freezer paper (for lining the mold)

Thermometer

Crockpot or double boiler

Instructions:

1. **Safety First:** Put on gloves and goggles to defend yourself while working with lye.

2. **Prepare the Lye Solution:**

Weigh out distilled water in a warmth-resistant container.

Carefully mixture inside the sodium hydroxide to the water in a certainly considered one of a type field. Do this in a properly-ventilated vicinity due to the fact the answer will heat up and emit fumes.

Allow the lye approach to cool to around a hundred and twenty°F (48°C) the usage of a thermometer.

three. Prepare the Oils:

In a warmth-resistant challenge, weigh out the coconut oil, olive oil, shea butter, and sunflower oil.

Shea butter and oils need to be melted collectively. Both a microwave and a double boiler are options.

4. Combine Lye Solution and Oils:

When every the lye solution and the oils have cooled to round 100 and twenty°F (48°C), slowly pour the lye solution into the melted oils.

Blend the contents with a stick blender till it reaches a mild trace. This shows that the combination has thickened to the point wherein a skinny trail, or "hint," is left inside the back of at the ground.

five. Hot Process in a Crockpot:

Transfer the soap aggregate to a crockpot set on low warmth.

Stir sometimes with a warm temperature-resistant spoon to save you sizzling.

6. Coconut Milk Addition:

Gently heat the canned coconut milk until it is at for the duration of the same temperature because the cleaning soap aggregate.

Slowly add the coconut milk to the cleansing cleaning soap inside the crockpot, stirring properly.

7. Cook and Monitor:

Cook the cleansing cleansing cleaning soap mixture inside the crockpot on low warmth, stirring sometimes.

The cleansing cleansing cleaning soap will undergo numerous tiers, along facet maintaining other than the edges of the crockpot and turning translucent.

eight. Testing for Doneness:

Perform a "zap" take a look at to check if the cleaning soap is steady to touch. Touch a small quantity of cleaning soap to your tongue. If it'd now not zap or tingle, the cleaning cleansing soap is stable.

You can also check for doneness with the resource of checking if the soap batter has a mashed potato-like consistency.

nine. Add Essential Oil and Colorant:

Once the cleansing cleansing cleaning soap is truely cooked and has reached the favored consistency, turn off the warm temperature.

Stir in your chosen critical oil and any natural colorants if desired.

10. Molding and Cooling:

Line your cleaning soap mould with parchment paper or freezer paper for smooth removal.

Spoon the cleansing soap batter into the mildew with warning, then use a spatula to clean the top.

For numerous hours or in a single day, permit the cleaning cleaning soap cool and corporation in the mold.

11. Cut and Cure:

Gently cast off the cleansing cleaning soap from the mildew as quickly because it has certainly cooled and employer, then slice it into bars.

Place the lessen bars on a drying rack to remedy for four-6 weeks. Due to the evaporation of additional water, the cleansing cleaning soap may also harden and grow to be milder as a end result.

12. Enjoy: After the curing period, your vegan coconut milk with shea butter cleaning cleansing soap is prepared for use and loved!

NEEM SOAP

Ingredients:

300g Coconut Oil

150g Olive Oil

150g Sunflower Oil

50g Shea Butter

100g Neem Oil

80g Sodium Hydroxide (Lye)

180g Distilled Water

10-15g Neem Leaf Powder (for coloration)

15-20g Essential Oil Blend (e.G., Tea Tree, Lavender)

Optional: Dried Neem Leaves for adornment

Tools:

Safety goggles, gloves, and apron

Digital kitchen scale

Stainless metal or warm temperature-resistant plastic blending bowls

Immersion blender

Thermometer

Silicone spatulas or timber spoons

Double boiler or microwave-stable box

Soap mould (silicone or wood)

Instructions:

1. Safety Precautions:

Put on your protection device, which incorporates goggles, gloves, and an apron.

Work in a nicely-ventilated place, away from children and pets.

2. Prepare the Lye Solution:

In a warmth-resistant field, measure the distilled water.

Gently whisk the water on the equal time as slowly incorporating the sodium hydroxide.

Place the lye answer in a constant place, far from any functionality dangers, and permit it to loosen up to round one hundred ten°F (40 three°C).

three. Prepare the Oils:

In a mixing bowl, tally the quantities of neem oil, shea butter, coconut oil, olive oil, and sunflower oil.

Use a double boiler or a microwave to melt the oils and butters till absolutely melted.

4. Mix the Lye Solution and Oils:

Make positive the lye solution and oils are both round a hundred and ten°F (43°C) in temperature.

Using an immersion blender to combine, lightly pour the lye answer into the oils.

Blend till best a tiny residue remains (just like a skinny cake batter consistency).

five. Cooking the Soap (Hot Process):

Transfer the cleansing cleaning cleaning soap combination to a warmth-resistant pot or slow cooker.

Set the pot over low warm temperature (if the use of a selection) or spark off the sluggish cooker to its lowest placing.

Stir the cleansing soap now and again as it chefs. It will undergo severa levels, emerge as translucent, and ultimately resemble mashed potatoes.

6. Checking for Doneness:

The cleaning cleaning soap is completed at the same time because it now not has any lye odor and has a clean texture (typically takes round 1-2 hours).

Test the cleansing cleansing cleaning soap through taking a small quantity and rubbing it amongst your gloved palms. If there is no zap (tingling sensation), it's prepared.

7. Adding Neem Leaf Powder and Essential Oils:

Once the cleaning soap is cooked, dispose of it from warm temperature.

Add neem leaf powder and vital oils to the cleaning cleaning soap, stirring nicely to distribute them evenly.

8. Molding and Decorating:

Use a silicone mildew or line your soap mould with parchment paper.

Carefully pour the cleaning soap into the mildew and easy the top with a spatula.

Press dried neem leaves onto the cleaning soap's top if you need to enhance it.

9. Curing:

Give the cleaning soap about 24 hours to kick back and solidify within the mould.

Unmold the cleaning cleaning soap after which slice it into bars.

For 4-6 weeks, region the bars on a curing rack in a fab, dry area with tremendous airflow. To acquire even drying, on occasion turn them.

10. Enjoy:

Once the curing period is whole, your vegan neem cleansing cleansing soap is ready to apply and experience.

Chapter 7: Melt & Pour Recipes

GRAPEFRUIT LEMON SOAP

Ingredients:

3 hundred grams clear melt and pour cleaning soap base

10 grams grapefruit vital oil

5 grams lemon vital oil

1 teaspoon dried lemon zest (for exfoliation)

Yellow cleansing soap colorant (herbal or mica-primarily based totally)

Soap-strong silicone mildew

Rubbing alcohol in a sprig bottle (for putting off air bubbles)

Tools:

Heat-consistent glass measuring cup

Microwave or double boiler

Mixing spoon or spatula

Kitchen scale (grams)

Knife or cleaning cleaning soap cutter

Instructions:

1. Prepare your workspace

Make positive your workspace is spotless and properly-prepared. Before starting, acquire all your additives and machine.

2. Cut Soap Base

Cut the clean soften and pour the cleansing soap base into small portions with a knife or cleansing cleaning soap cutter. This promotes even melting.

3. Melt Soap Base

Place the cleansing soap chunks in a warmth-steady glass measuring cup. In the microwave, soften the cleaning cleaning soap base for the duration of durations of 15 to 30 seconds, stirring in among. As an possibility, you will in all likelihood use a stovetop double boiler.

4. Add Essential Oils and Colorant

Once the cleansing cleaning soap base is truely melted, upload the grapefruit and lemon critical oils. Mix well to ensure even distribution. Add a small quantity of yellow cleaning cleaning soap colorant till to procure the preferred colour. Stir till the colour is uniform.

5. Add Exfoliant

Sprinkle the dried lemon zest into the cleaning cleaning soap aggregate. The zest gives a mild exfoliating impact and complements the citrus heady scent. Stir gently to distribute the zest.

6. Pour into Mold

Pour the scented and coloured cleaning cleaning soap mixture into the cleaning soap-stable silicone mould. Gently tap the mildew on the counter to release any air bubbles. If bubbles stay at the floor, spritz the top of the cleaning soap with rubbing alcohol to get rid of them.

7. Allow to Cool and Solidify

For some hours, permit the cleansing cleaning soap cool and organization inside the mould. To hasten the cooling machine, you may moreover located the mold in the refrigerator.

8. Unmold and Cut

Once the cleansing cleaning soap is clearly cooled and sturdy, carefully pop it out of the mildew. Use a knife or cleaning cleaning soap cutter to slice the cleansing soap into individual bars.

nine. Allow Curing

Place the lessen bars on a smooth and dry surface to remedy for about 24 - forty eight hours. During this time, the soap hardens, and any extra moisture evaporates.

10. Ready for Use

After curing, your Grapefruit Lemon cleaning cleaning soap is prepared to be used or gifting. Store the cleansing soap in a cool, dry location to preserve its freshness.

Enjoy the fresh citrus perfume and exfoliating homes of your natural Grapefruit Lemon cleaning soap!

REFRESHING GERANIUM SOAP

Ingredients:

hundred grams easy melt and pour cleaning soap base

1 teaspoon geranium crucial oil

1 teaspoon spirulina powder (for colour)

Dried rose petals (for decoration)

Tools:

Heat-secure container or microwave-solid bowl

Cutting board

Soap mildew (silicone molds paintings well)

Stirring utensil (stainless-steel or warmth-resistant plastic)

Spray bottle full of rubbing alcohol (to do away with air bubbles)

Digital kitchen scale

Instructions:

1. Prepare Workspace:

Clean and sanitize all tool and workspace to make certain a hygienic cleansing soap-making method.

Set up your cleaning cleaning soap mildew on a flat floor for smooth pouring.

2. Cut Soap Base:

Cut the clean soften and pour cleansing cleaning soap base into small cubes the usage of a pointy knife and a clean decreasing board. This promotes even cleaning soap melting.

three. Melt Soap Base:

In a basin or box that may be carried out in a microwave, located the cleaning soap cubes.

In the microwave, soften the cleansing cleansing soap cubes in 20-2nd periods, stirring after every one to make certain complete melting. Alternatively, you'll in all likelihood use a stovetop double boiler.

four. Add Geranium Essential Oil:

Remove the cleaning cleaning soap base from the heat supply as quickly as it has really melted.

Add 1 teaspoon of geranium critical oil to the melted cleaning soap base. Stir lightly to distribute the oil evenly.

5. Add Color:

To the melted cleaning cleaning soap base, upload 1 teaspoon of geranium essential oil. This will supply your cleansing soap a easy inexperienced color. Adjust the amount of colorant for your desired shade.

Stir the cleansing soap base until the colour is properly covered.

6. Prepare Mold:

Place the cleaning soap mildew on a strong floor.

Lightly spray the internal of the mould cavities with rubbing alcohol. This lets in to put off air bubbles.

7. Pour Soap Base:

Slowly pour the coloured cleansing soap base into the mould cavities. Pour slowly and from a low pinnacle to limit the formation of air bubbles.

eight. Spritz with Rubbing Alcohol:

Immediately after pouring the cleansing cleansing cleaning soap, lightly spritz the ground of the cleansing cleaning cleaning soap in every hollow space with rubbing alcohol. This allows to pop any last air bubbles.

9. Add Dried Rose Petals:

While the cleaning soap remains really gentle, gently area dried rose petals on the ground of each cleaning soap hole area. Press the petals barely to stick them to the cleansing cleaning soap.

10. Allow to Set:

For several hours, or till the cleaning cleaning soap is completely stiffened, permit it cool and solidify in the mildew. Depending on the dimensions of your cleaning cleansing cleaning soap bars, this may take anywhere from one to 4 hours.

eleven. Unmold and Enjoy:

Gently press at the all over again of the mould whilst the cleansing cleansing soap has completely cooled and hardened to launch the cleaning cleaning soap bars.

Your Refreshing Geranium Soap is now geared up to use or as a gift!

ROSEMARY CITRUS SOAP

Ingredients:

200 grams clean glycerin melt-and-pour cleaning cleansing cleaning soap base

10 grams rosemary-infused olive oil (or easy olive oil)

5 grams candy almond oil

five grams grapefruit essential oil

2 grams rosemary crucial oil

Dried rosemary leaves (for exfoliation and ornament)

Natural colorants (optional): Spirulina powder (green), turmeric powder (yellow), paprika powder (orange)

Tools:

Microwave-solid glass measuring cup or double boiler

Stirring utensil (plastic or silicone)

Soap mildew (silicone molds work nicely)

Spray bottle complete of rubbing alcohol (for putting off air bubbles)

Instructions:

1. Prepare Ingredients:

To facilitate melting, chop the easy glycerin melt-and-pour cleansing soap base into doable portions.

Measure the candy almond oil, rosemary crucial oil, grapefruit important oil, and olive oil infused with rosemary.

2. Melt Soap Base:

Put the cleaning cleaning cleaning soap chunks in a double boiler or a tumbler measuring cup that may be used in the microwave.

Melt the cleansing soap base withIn the double boiler or in 20 to 30 2nd intervals over low warm temperature in the microwave. To ensure complete melting, stir continuously.

three. Add Oils and Essential Oils:

Once the soap base is melted, upload the rosemary-infused olive oil and sweet almond oil. Stir to mix.

Allow the cleaning cleaning soap mixture to cool barely earlier than including the critical oils to hold their fragrance.

four. Add Essential Oils:

Add the grapefruit crucial oil and rosemary essential oil to the cleansing cleaning soap combination. Stir gently to distribute the oils lightly.

five. Optional: Add Colorants:

If you'd like to function a touch of shade, you may use natural colorants like spirulina powder, turmeric powder, or paprika powder. Start with a small pinch of the preferred powder and stir well. Adjust the quantity till you acquire the preferred hue.

6. Pour Soap into Mold:

Sprinkle a tiny quantity of dried rosemary leaves into the cleansing cleansing cleaning soap molds if you need to apply them as an exfoliant and adornment.

Pour the melted cleaning cleaning soap aggregate into the cleaning soap mould steadily (s). Each cavity want to be nearly complete, with some room very last.

7. Spritz with Rubbing Alcohol:

Spray a small mist of rubbing alcohol on the cleaning cleaning soap's ground to dispose of any air bubbles that can have developed at some level in the pouring approach.

8. Allow to Set:

Give the cleaning soap time to sit back and solidify inside the mildew, ideally for numerous hours.

nine. Unmold and Cut:

Gently pop the cleaning cleaning soap bars out of the molds. If you used dried rosemary leaves, they ought to be visible at the floor of the cleansing soap.

If preferred, you could now reduce the soap bars into your preferred length and form.

10. Curing:

Melt and pour cleaning cleaning soap does now not require the same curing time as bloodless-technique soap. You can use your rosemary citrus cleaning cleaning soap inner a few hours of unmolding.

Chapter 8: Lemon Pumice Soap

Ingredients:

300 grams Clear Melt and Pour Soap Base

10 grams Pumice Powder

10 grams Lemon Essential Oil

Lemon Zest (from 1-2 lemons)

Yellow Soap Colorant (optionally to be had)

Tools:

Microwave or Double Boiler

Heat-secure box

Soap mold (silicone molds work nicely)

Mixing spoon or spatula

Knife or cleansing cleansing soap cutter

Instructions:

1. Prepare Your Workspace: Set up your workspace with all of the vital tools and factors. Ensure your cleansing cleaning

cleaning soap mould is easy and ready for use.

2. Cut Soap Base: Cut three hundred grams of smooth melt and pour cleansing cleansing cleaning soap base into small chunks. This permits the cleansing soap melt lightly.

three. Melt Soap Base: Place the cleansing cleaning cleaning soap chunks in a heat-steady field. Use the microwave to step by step melt the cleansing cleaning soap base at 15-20 2nd durations, stirring in amongst. As an possibility, you could soften subjects in a double boiler.

four. Add Lemon Zest: Once the soap base is honestly melted, add the lemon zest to the melted cleaning cleaning soap. The zest gives a herbal contact and seen enchantment to the cleaning cleaning soap.

five. Add Pumice Powder: Mix in 10 grams of pumice powder into the melted cleaning cleaning soap. Pumice is a herbal exfoliant that adds texture to the cleaning soap, making it excellent for doing away with vain pores and pores and skin cells.

6. Add Lemon Essential Oil: Stir in 10 grams of lemon crucial oil for a easy citrus perfume. Lemon critical oil is also referred to for its cleaning and invigorating homes.

7. Add Soap Colorant (Optional): If you want to beautify the yellow shade of the cleansing cleansing cleaning soap, you could add a small quantity of yellow cleansing soap colorant. Always keep in thoughts that a bit goes an prolonged way, so begin with a small drop and make changes as essential.

eight. Mix Thoroughly: Stir the combination very well to lightly distribute the zest, pumice, essential oil, and colorant (if used). Make great all of the materials are properly covered.

9. Pour into Mold: Carefully pour the cleaning soap mixture into your cleansing cleaning soap mildew. If you need a layered impact, pour a small quantity, permit it cool and in

detail solidify, after which pour the ultimate cleansing cleansing soap on top.

10. Cool and Solidify: Allow the cleansing cleaning soap to relax and solidify within the mould. This generally takes a couple of hours, but the perfect time can also range.

eleven. Unmold and Cut: Gently dispose of the cleansing cleaning soap from the mildew as quick because it has absolutely cooled and solidified. To lessen the cleansing cleaning cleaning soap into bars of the specified period, use a knife or cleaning cleaning soap cutter.

12. Curing: Put the reduce bars on a drying rack or tray and permit them to some days to remedy. This ensures a cleaning soap bar so one can remaining longer by using permitting any extra moisture to get away.

13. Labeling and Storage: Once truly cured, label your Lemon Pumice Soap with the components and date. Store the cleaning

soap in a fab, dry place or wrap it in wax paper to hold its freshness.

Chapter 9: The Essence Of Vegan Soap Crafting

In "DIY Soap Making for Vegans: Crafting Luscious Vegan Soaps," we've got released right into a journey that transcends the mere act of cleansing cleaning soap making. It's a symphony of scents, shades, textures, and values, all coming collectively to create herbal, plant-powered pampering testimonies. In this economic smash, we are going to delve deeper into the very middle of what makes crafting vegan soaps this form of splendid and fun mission.

Exploring the Art of Vegan Soap Making

As we step into the world of crafting vegan soaps, we discover ourselves at the intersection of era and creativity. Imagine yourself as every a chemist and an artist, wielding herbal oils, butters, and fragrances as your system. It's now not genuinely cleaning cleaning soap you're developing; it's far a bit of art work.

At the coronary heart of this progressive approach is the fascinating concept of saponification, wherein oils and an alkaline solution react to shape cleansing soap and glycerin. This chemical transformation underpins each cleaning soap bar you craft. Understanding the chemistry in the back of cleansing cleaning soap making empowers you to tailor your creations to perfection.

In this financial disaster, we'll find out the technological know-how of soap making in extra element, demystifying the saponification technique. You'll advantage insights into the residences of severa oils and butters, permitting you to pick out factors that cater on your pores and skin's unique needs. Whether you are aiming for a wealthy, moisturizing cleaning soap or one with a costly lather, we will manual you thru the art work of aspect choice.

Understanding the Whys and Hows

Now, permit's pause to ponder the "why" inside the lower back of your preference of vegan cleansing soap making. It's now not merely about crafting cleaning soap; it is about embracing a holistic manner of existence that champions each private well-being and worldwide concord. Here, we are able to delve into critical factors:

1. Skin-Friendly Goodness: Vegan cleansing soap is a address for your pores and pores and skin. Free from animal fat and merciless chemical compounds, it is slight and nourishing. We'll delve into the advantages of using vegan cleansing cleansing soap, from alleviating skin problems to selling state-of-the-art pores and pores and skin fitness.

2. Cruelty-Free Compassion: Your desire of vegan cleaning soap extends past self-care; it's an moral stance. By eschewing animal-derived components and cruelty, you are contributing to a greater compassionate international. We'll delve into the ethics of vegan cleaning cleaning soap making, discussing the significance of respecting animal welfare.

three. Environmental Responsibility: Vegan cleansing soap is an eco-aware choice. It reduces your ecological footprint with the aid of warding off the environmental effect associated with animal agriculture. We'll find out how your cleansing cleansing soap-making choices can align with environmental stewardship.

4. Artistic Expression: Vegan cleansing cleansing soap making is a revolutionary outlet. Just as a painter selects shades and brushes, you may pick oils, fragrances, and designs to craft unique cleansing cleansing soap bars that mirror your fashion and individual. We'll talk the manner to tap into your creativity and create signature soap recipes.

5. Community and Sharing: Crafting vegan soaps isn't just a solitary pursuit; it's far an possibility to connect to like-minded human beings. We'll discover how you may be a part of cleaning cleaning soap-making groups,

percent your creations, and inspire others to embody this enriching journey.

By the stop of this financial ruin, you may have obtained a deeper expertise of the art work and technology of vegan cleansing cleansing soap making. You'll be geared up with the information to choose out materials that align collectively together with your pores and pores and skin's desires, ethical values, and environmental worries. As you continue to find out the place of crafting luscious vegan soaps, don't forget that it's miles no longer pretty a lot growing soap; it's far approximately nurturing a holistic way of lifestyles that celebrates splendor, compassion, and sustainability.

Essential Tools and Equipment

In our journey via "DIY Soap Making for Vegans: Crafting Luscious Vegan Soaps," we've got got explored the creative and ethical dimensions of vegan cleansing cleansing cleaning soap crafting. Now, it's time to get sensible. In this bankruptcy, we are going to delve into the essential gadget and device you can want to embark in your cleansing soap-making journey, putting you up for fulfillment inside the worldwide of plant-powered pampering.

Gathering Your Soap-Making Arsenal

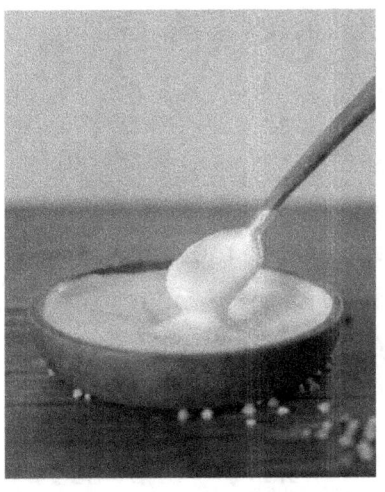

Before you could create your first vegan cleaning soap masterpiece, you may want to supply collectively your cleansing cleaning soap-making toolkit. Think of it as your cleansing cleaning soap-making laboratory, filled with gadgets that allow you to remodel uncooked substances into pricey cleansing cleansing soap bars. Let's take a higher take a look at what those gadgets are and why they'll be important:

1. Mixing Bowls: You'll need numerous blending bowls to mix your factors. These should be robust, smooth to clean, and distinct absolutely for soap making to avoid infection.

2. Stirring Tools: Wooden or silicone spatulas and whisks are your excellent buddies in the cleaning soap-making method. They need to be long lasting, warm temperature-resistant, and non-reactive with the cleaning soap substances.

3. Molds: Soap molds are to be had in severa styles and sizes, allowing you to get cutting-edge alongside aspect your cleansing cleansing cleaning soap designs. We'll talk remarkable styles of molds and a way to choose the proper ones to your tasks.

4. Thermometers: Precision subjects in cleansing soap making, and an awesome thermometer permits you reveal the temperature of your additives as it should be.

5. Safety Gear: This consists of gadgets like gloves and safety goggles to shield your self at some stage in the cleansing cleaning soap-making approach.

6. Scale: A virtual kitchen scale is treasured for specific measuring of things.

7. Containers: You'll want packing containers to store and diploma your oils, lye, and brilliant elements.

eight. Soap Cutter: A dedicated cleaning cleaning cleaning soap cutter permits you purchased clean, even cuts while your cleaning cleansing soap is ready to be sliced into bars.

9. Immersion Blender: While now not compulsory, an immersion blender can simplify the mixture approach, specially for more complex soap recipes.

We'll no longer excellent speak the middle components of your cleansing cleansing soap-making device however moreover emphasize the significance of selecting the right substances. Ensuring that your tools are crafted from substances that may not react with the cleaning cleaning soap materials or compromise their tremendous is crucial.

Moreover, we're going to offer pointers on where to deliver those equipment and the way to attend to them to lengthen their lifespan, making your funding in cleaning cleaning soap-making device worthwhile.

Setting Up Your Soap-Making Space

Now which you have your equipment in hand, it is time to set the degree in your soap-making creations. Your cleaning cleaning soap-making region should be organized, properly-ventilated, and equipped to cope with functionality spills and messes.

1. Organization: A nicely-prepared workspace is critical for a easy cleansing cleaning soap-

making system. We'll guide you via setting up your cleaning soap-making region, ensuring that the entirety is inner reach.

2. Ventilation: Proper air glide is important whilst running with high quality factors, collectively with lye. We'll speak a way to create a suitable environment that allows for top air flow into and minimizes exposure to fumes.

3. Safety Measures: Safety is a top priority in cleansing cleaning soap making. We'll discover ways to guard your self, which encompass the use of protection goggles, gloves, and aprons. Additionally, we're going to offer steerage on what to do in case of unintentional spills or touch with soap-making substances.

4. Surface Protection: Soap making can be messy. We'll provide pointers on a way to guard your work surfaces, whether or not you are strolling in a kitchen or a devoted cleaning cleaning soap-making area.

5. Cleaning and Maintenance: Keeping your cleansing cleaning soap-making location clean is not simplest vital for hygiene but moreover extends the life of your tool. We'll proportion quality practices for cleaning up after each cleaning cleaning cleaning soap-making consultation and retaining your device.

As we development thru this entire bankruptcy, you may advantage a deep understanding of the gear and surroundings essential for your vegan cleaning cleaning cleaning soap-making endeavors. With your cleansing cleaning soap-making arsenal and workspace in order, you'll be well-organized to dive into the palms-on factors of crafting your non-public vegan soaps in the upcoming chapters. Get prepared to transform your additives into delightful bars of vegan goodness.

Chapter 10: Vegan Soap Recipes

In our adventure thru "DIY Soap Making for Vegans: Crafting Luscious Vegan Soaps," we've got were given had been given laid the muse, exploring the artwork and technological information of vegan cleansing cleaning soap crafting and information the essence of this extraordinary enterprise. Now, it is time to roll up your sleeves, acquire your components, and immerse your self in the hands-on worldwide of cleansing cleaning soap making. This financial disaster is your gateway to growing vegan cleansing cleaning soap masterpieces that allows you to pride your senses and pamper your pores and pores and skin.

Basic Vegan Soap Recipe

We'll begin with a crucial vegan cleaning soap recipe, a canvas upon which you may explicit your creativity and craft personalised soaps. This foundational recipe will introduce you to the middle ideas of soap making, from measuring and mixing components to achieving the favored cleansing cleansing cleaning soap consistency. You'll learn how to integrate plant-primarily based oils, lye, and water in precise portions to initiate the paranormal gadget of saponification.

As we guide you via this recipe, we're going to emphasize the significance of safety measures, temperature manage, and proper blending strategies. By the forestall of this phase, you will have produced your first batch of vegan cleansing cleaning soap, a second of accomplishment and a testament in your budding cleaning cleaning soap-making skills.

Customizing Your Soap: Fragrances and Colors

With the fundamentals below your belt, we are going to dive deeper into the arena of customization. One of the thrill of soap making is the capability to infuse your creations with exceptional fragrances and beautiful colors. Here, we can discover those innovative dimensions of cleansing cleaning soap crafting:

Fragrances: Essential oils are your olfactory palette, providing an array of scents, from soothing lavender to invigorating citrus. We'll provide steering on choosing essential oils, mixing fragrances, and challenge the right heady scent balance on your cleansing soap. Discover how aromatherapy and cleaning cleaning soap making intertwine to create no longer only a cleansing revel in however a sensory adventure.

Colors: Nature offers a colourful spectrum of colours that may be harnessed to add seen appeal on your soaps. We'll delve into natural colorants, along with herbs, spices, and clays, which now not first-class tint your soaps but additionally infuse them with extra pores and skin-loving houses. If you're on the lookout for extra vibrant colorings, we'll discover steady synthetic shade alternatives that open up a international of opportunities in your cleansing soap designs.

Throughout this financial ruin, you may discover exceptional commands for crafting diverse cleaning soap recipes, each supplying a completely particular mixture of fragrances and colours. Whether you are developing a relaxing lavender-scented cleansing cleaning soap with smooth pastel shades or an energizing citrus explosion with ambitious, colorful colorings, you may have the gadget and facts to supply your cleaning cleansing cleaning soap-making visions to life.

As you development via the recipes, endure in thoughts that cleaning soap making is every a technology and an paintings. Each batch is an possibility to experiment, refine your strategies, and develop your signature soap-making fashion. By the surrender of this financial catastrophe, you can now not fine have a fixed of beautiful vegan soaps but additionally the self guarantee to discover extra advanced strategies and designs in the chapters that observe.

Get prepared to immerse your self in the worldwide of vegan cleansing cleaning cleaning soap creation, wherein your creativity is aware of no bounds, and each bar of soap becomes a canvas on your creative expression.

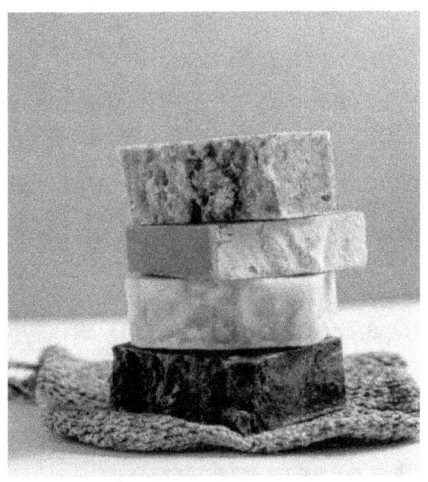

Advanced Techniques

In the world of "DIY Soap Making for Vegans: Crafting Luscious Vegan Soaps," we have were given got ventured past the basics and explored the artwork of crafting cute vegan soaps. Now, it is time to raise your cleansing cleaning soap making skills further and embark on a adventure into the world of superior techniques. This chapter is your gateway to growing brilliant cleansing cleansing cleaning soap designs so one can not best cleanse but moreover captivate the senses.

Layered and Swirled Soaps

Imagine cleaning cleansing cleaning soap bars with complex layers of colors and swirls that resemble works of art. Layered and swirled soaps are not best visually lovable however moreover provide a sensorial enjoy like no certainly one of a kind. In this segment, we're going to manual you through the manner of creating the ones fascinating soap designs.

You'll have a look at techniques for pouring and layering cleansing soap batter to acquire great strata of colors and textures. We'll additionally delve into the paintings of swirling, wherein you could create enchanting styles via lightly manipulating the cleansing soap's ground. From sensitive pastel gradients to bold, contrasting swirls, you may discover countless possibilities for expressing your creativity.

Embeds and Inclusions

Elevate your cleaning cleaning soap designs further through incorporating embeds and inclusions. These are like hidden treasures indoors your cleansing cleaning cleaning soap bars, which includes intrigue and surprise to every use. We'll find out the region of embeds and inclusions, allowing you to infuse your soaps with extra factors of beauty and capability.

Embeds: These are small cleaning soap creations which is probably embedded internal a bigger cleansing cleansing soap bar. You can craft mini cleansing cleaning soap shapes, colorful cubes, or perhaps embed dried flowers for a touch of herbal beauty. We'll manual you thru the gadget of making and putting embeds to acquire lovely visible results.

Inclusions: Inclusions are gadgets or elements delivered to cleaning cleaning soap for his or her beneficial or aesthetic price. From exfoliating components like oatmeal and poppy seeds to botanical factors like dried herbs and petals, you could discover ways to include the ones enhancements into your soap recipes. Each inclusion brings precise advantages, reworking your cleansing soap bars into multi-dimensional memories.

Shaping and Molding Techniques

Step into the location of specific soap shapes and molds, in which you could craft cleaning soap bars that stand proud of the ordinary. We'll discover various shaping and molding strategies that will let you create cleansing cleaning soap in fantastic workplace work and sizes.

You'll find out the manner to apply robust point molds to craft cleansing soap in shapes starting from delicate hearts and plants to complex geometrics and summary designs. Additionally, we are going to manual you thru the device of hand-molding cleaning soap, supplying you the freedom to create certainly one-of-a-kind cleaning cleansing soap creations that replicate your personality and fashion.

Throughout this economic break, you will locate particular instructions for superior cleaning cleaning soap recipes that incorporate these strategies. Whether you are designing layered and swirled soaps harking back to ocean waves, embedding colorful cleaning soap gems, or crafting cleaning cleaning soap bars in particular styles and sizes, you could have the know-how and abilties to push the boundaries of your cleaning cleaning soap-making artistry.

Remember that advanced cleansing soap making is an invite to unleash your creativity absolutely. Each cleansing cleaning soap creation becomes a masterpiece, a testomony to your evolving skills and creative vision. By the cease of this financial disaster, you'll no longer handiest have an array of lovely vegan soaps however additionally the self belief to discover even more difficult and resourceful cleaning soap designs inside the chapters that comply with.

Prepare to be surprised as you dive into the arena of superior cleaning cleansing soap techniques, wherein the first-rate restriction is your imagination, and each cleaning cleaning soap bar will become a bit of art that tells a story of know-how and creativity.

Chapter 11: Troubleshooting And Common Pitfalls

In "DIY Soap Making for Vegans: Crafting Luscious Vegan Soaps," we've got launched into a adventure into the fascinating global of crafting vegan soaps. By now, you have got explored the basics, created adorable cleansing cleaning soap designs, and ventured into superior techniques. Yet, as with all craft, worrying situations can also upward thrust up alongside the way. This financial disaster is your manual to troubleshooting commonplace problems and pitfalls in cleansing cleaning soap making, ensuring that your cleansing cleaning cleaning soap creations live a supply of pride and delight.

Addressing Common Soap-Making Challenges

Soap making, like every creative employer, comes with its percentage of traumatic conditions. Whether you're a newbie or an professional cleansing cleaning soap crafter, it's far crucial to understand a manner to tackle not unusual problems that can upward push up sooner or later of the cleaning soap-making machine. In this segment, we are able to cope with the ones demanding conditions and offer solutions:

1. Acceleration or Seizing: Sometimes, cleaning cleaning soap batter can boost up or capture suddenly, making it difficult to art work with. We'll discover the reasons in the back of the ones issues and percentage techniques to regain manage and salvage your soap batch.

2. Soda Ash: Soda ash is a harmless however unpleasant white powder that would shape at the surface of cleansing cleaning soap. We'll speak preventive measures and removal techniques to preserve your cleaning cleaning soap bars pristine.

three. Discoloration: Soap colors can also shift or trade over the years because of different factors. You'll learn how to assume and control discoloration, making sure your cleansing cleaning cleaning soap maintains its intended appearance.

4. Scent Fading: Fragrances can every so often fade as cleaning cleaning soap treatments. We'll percent guidelines for selecting strong scents and techniques to maintain the aromatic appeal of your soaps.

five. Cracking or Splitting: Soap bars can also broaden cracks or splits in some unspecified time in the future of curing. We'll manual you on stopping those structural problems and keeping the integrity of your cleansing soap creations.

Preventing and Fixing Mistakes

Mistakes are a herbal a part of any gaining knowledge of machine, and cleaning cleaning soap making is not any exception. This phase will assist you navigate through mishaps and offer insights into prevention and correction:

1. Lye Safety: Safety is paramount in cleaning soap making, and we are able to reiterate the significance of proper handling and storage of lye to keep away from accidents.

2. Batch Rebatching: If a cleansing cleansing cleaning soap batch does not flip out as deliberate, rebatching lets in you to salvage and rework it into usable cleaning cleaning cleaning soap. We'll provide step-with the aid of-step commands in this valuable technique.

3. Recycling Soap Scraps: Don't allow leftover cleaning soap scraps go to waste. Learn a way to recycle and reshape them into new cleansing soap bars, reducing waste and saving property.

four. Storing and Curing: Properly storing and curing your cleansing cleaning soap is important for its first-class and durability. We'll percentage splendid practices to ensure your cleansing cleaning soap stays in pinnacle situation.

By the end of this chapter, you will have a complete information of the manner to troubleshoot and triumph over not unusual stressful conditions that can rise up within the route of your cleansing cleaning soap-making journey. Whether you are dealing with sudden acceleration, soda ash, discoloration, fragrance fading, or structural troubles like cracking, you may be nicely-equipped to address the ones problems with self assurance.

Remember, making errors is an essential a part of mastering any craft. With the insights and answers supplied in this financial catastrophe, you can not fine troubleshoot effectively however moreover turn mishaps into possibilities for increase and creativity.

In addition to addressing challenges, we are able to deliver a lift to the significance of lye protection, ensuring which you manipulate this crucial soap-making factor with care and precision.

Furthermore, you can discover the artwork of batch rebatching, a precious technique that permits you to rescue cleaning cleaning soap batches that failed to flow as planned. Turn the ones batches into specific creations that showcase your adaptability as a cleaning soap maker.

But it'd no longer save you there. We'll additionally show you a way to make the maximum of each cleansing soap beneficial useful resource, from recycling soap scraps to proper storage and curing practices, making sure that your cleaning cleaning soap creations live colourful and extended-lasting.

So, as you navigate the arena of cleansing cleaning soap making, recollect that disturbing situations are clearly stepping stones on your path to cleaning cleaning soap-making mastery. Embrace the troubleshooting abilties you obtain in this economic ruin, and permit your creativity shine thru every cleaning soap advent.

Now, permit's flow in advance with self belief, information that no cleaning soap-making obstacle can stand in the way of your journey to crafting luscious vegan soaps.

Vegan Ingredients for Extra Pampering

In "DIY Soap Making for Vegans: Crafting Luscious Vegan Soaps," we have were given traversed the fascinating panorama of cleaning soap crafting, from the important fundamentals to advanced techniques and troubleshooting. Now, it's time to delve deeper into the place of vegan cleaning cleaning soap factors, in which you may find out a treasure trove of herbal elements that would increase your cleaning cleaning soap creations to new heights of pampering and indulgence.

Exploring Specialty Oils and Butters

One of the defining traits of vegan soaps is the use of plant-based completely oils and butters, each with its precise homes and benefits. In this section, we're going to embark on a adventure thru a lush garden of oils and butters which can beautify the best of your cleaning soap:

Coconut Oil: Renowned for its adequate lather and cleansing capabilities, coconut oil is a cleaning cleaning soap-making staple. We'll discover its role in soap formulations and its impact at the completed product.

Olive Oil: Olive oil brings a hint of steeply-priced on your cleaning cleaning soap bars, supplying mildness and moisturization. Discover how to encompass this timeless thing into your cleansing cleaning soap recipes.

Shea Butter: Shea butter is a rich, creamy butter that imparts nourishment and hydration to the skin. We'll delve into its skin care benefits and strategies for the usage of it in soap making.

Avocado Oil: Avocado oil is a supply of nutrients and antioxidants, making it an incredible preference for pores and skin-amazing soaps. Learn a manner to harness its houses to create moisturizing cleansing soap bars.

www.ingramcontent.com/pod-product-compliance
Lightning Source LLC
Chambersburg PA
CBHW071447080526
44587CB00014B/2017